THE LITTLE
STRENGTH
TRAINING
BOOK

THE LITTLE
STRENGTH TRAINING
BOOK

ERIKA DILLMAN

WARNER BOOKS

An AOL Time Warner Company

Neither these exercises and programs nor any other exercise program should be followed without first consulting a health care professional. If you have any special conditions requiring attention, you should consult with your health care professional regularly regarding possible modifications of the program contained in this book.

Copyright © 2004 by Erika Dillman
All rights reserved.

Warner Books, Inc., 1271 Avenue of the Americas, New York, NY 10020

Visit our Web site at www.twbookmark.com

 An AOL Time Warner Company

The *Little Strength Training Book*™ is part of the "Little Book" series owned by Warner Books. All rights to the series and the trade dress is the property of Warner Books, Inc.

Printed in the United States of America
First Printing: January 2004
10 9 8 7 6 5 4 3 2 1

ISBN: 0-446-69123-2

Library of Congress Control Number 2003048581

Book design and text composition by L&G McRee
Cover design by Rachel McClain
Text illustrations by Emma Vokurka

For Maddie

Acknowledgments

Thanks to the many people who contributed to *The Little Strength Training Book*:

My agent, Anne Depue; my editor, Diana Baroni, and assistant editor, Molly Chehak; and my friends and family for their continued support.

Emma Vokurka, for her wonderful illustrations.

Debby Heath, Stephanie Molliconi, Janet Clark, Ted Johnson, Suzan Huney, Jill Irwin, Anita McEntyre, and Seanna Brow for their helpful comments, suggestions, and proofreading.

And the many health and fitness experts who generously shared their time and expertise with me: William J. Kraemer, professor of exercise physiology, University of Connecticut;

ACKNOWLEDGMENTS

Wayne Wescott, Ph.D., fitness research director at the South Shore YMCA, Quincy, Massachusetts; Darcy Norman, physical therapist, certified athletic trainer, certified strength and conditioning specialist (CSCS); Michael Porter, M.S., health and fitness instructor (certified by the American College of Sports Medicine), CSCS; and C.C. Cunningham, M.S. certified athletic trainer, CSCS, and personal trainer (certified by the American Council on Exercise).

Contents

CONTENTS

THE LITTLE
STRENGTH TRAINING
BOOK

Welcome to *The Little Strength Training Book*

A NEW LOOK AT STRENGTH TRAINING

Strength training is a lot like eating more vegetables: it's good for you, but perhaps you haven't quite gotten into the habit yet. Maybe you think it'll take too much time, or you don't want to join a gym, or you're afraid that you'll end up looking like the Incredible Hulk.

On the other hand, wouldn't it be nice to be able to lift those economy-size bottles of laundry detergent without hurting yourself? And have more energy—not to mention, lose a few pounds, firm up the flab under your upper arms, and lower your blood pressure, all while increasing your stamina?

If you like the idea of having a stronger, healthier body, don't let a few misconceptions stand in your way. Strength training doesn't require a big time commitment; it can be done safely at home by people of all ages and abilities, and it will give you a stronger, firmer body without bulking you up. Fitness professionals recommend it as an essential component of a balanced fitness plan, along with aerobic and flexibility exercises.

How to Use This Book

Before practicing any of the exercises in this book, please read the preceding chapters to become more familiar with basic anatomy and physiology, body mechanics, strength training guidelines, and training techniques and tips. You will learn the importance of progressing gradually, mastering basic moves before taking on more challenging exercises. Learning the "how tos" and "whys" of strength training before practicing any of the exercises will help you get the most out of your workouts.

Welcome to *The Little Strength Training Book*

Whether you're a beginner or a frequent exerciser, you'll find this book easy to use. All of the exercises are described in step-by-step, easy-to-follow instructions, with no confusing sports jargon or hype.

I hope that in reading *The Little Strength Training Book* you not only learn how to master the exercises but also enjoy practicing them. With a small time commitment and consistent training, you will soon benefit from more energy and a stronger, leaner body.

ERIKA DILLMAN

1 | 135-Pound Weakling

WATER WEIGHT

I haven't exactly had sand kicked in my face, but I have experienced the independent woman's equivalent: having to ask my boyfriend to replace the five-gallon water jugs on my water dispenser.

For years, we had a perfect system. I wanted a drink; he did the heavy lifting. But when things got shaky between us, I was forced to take responsibility for my bottled water habit. First, I tried three-gallon jugs, but they were still too heavy for me to carry up to my second-floor apartment. Then, for a while,

I bought liter-size bottles of water. That didn't work either (too many trips to the store). Finally, faced with the prospect of having to drink tap water for the rest of my life, I decided to do something about my matchstick arms and rubbery torso.

CHANGING PERCEPTIONS

It's not like strength training was a mystery to me. I'd lifted weights in high school to prepare for the track season, although I rarely stuck with it once the season ended. Knowing I was in excellent cardiovascular shape from all the miles I logged, I had occasionally wondered whether lifting weights did anything for me but fatigue my already overworked muscles.

Even in my mid-twenties, when illness and injury prevented me from running, I still didn't consider lifting weights as a necessary part of my fitness routine. I wasn't "in training" for competition, my heart and lungs were in good shape, and I burned a lot of calories from swimming, walking, and biking. There were strong people and weak people, and I accepted that I was skinny and weak and always would be. I liked being thin. It worked for me. That is, until I hit my thirties and realized that I no longer had the body of an active sixteen-year-old.

Ten pounds overweight and lumpy in places I wanted to be firm, it wasn't only my struggles with oversize water jugs that caused me to take a fresh look at getting stronger. It had begun to seem like everyone was in shape but me. Sure, I wanted to lift my own bottles and carry my own suitcase. But I also wanted to look great in a little black dress.

STRENGTH, ENERGY, AND GRACE

I started working with a personal trainer at my health club who designed a few different strength training routines for me, each consisting of six or seven exercises to train all of the major muscle groups in my body. I started off with twice-a-week, twenty-to-thirty-minute workouts that I could do at home with no equipment or with handheld weights.

Initially, I worked with very light weights—only three- and five- pounders. Approaching each exercise like a yoga pose, I concentrated on using correct form, maintaining my posture, and coordinating my movement with my breath. Before each lift I inhaled slowly, focusing my mind on the task ahead, and as I lifted the weight, I exhaled slowly, controlling the pace with my breath. Then, inhaling slowly, I returned the weight to the starting position. I was surprised by how much I enjoyed the discipline and control required in strength training. It felt good to develop a rhythm that made me feel graceful and strong at the same time. My workouts left me feeling solid and energized, like I'd accomplished something important. Over time, I was able to gradually increase the amount of weight I lifted.

INDEPENDENCE RESTORED

Within a few months, my arms and legs felt firmer and had more muscle definition. Even my abs felt harder when I pressed on them. My trainer had assured me that I wouldn't bulk up from strength training, but rather firm up. She was right. I felt better, I looked better, and I started to notice other changes in my body. My coordination and balance improved. And I could walk farther before becoming fatigued.

It was still a bit challenging hauling those water jugs up two flights of stairs to my apartment, but I didn't throw out my back in the process and was strong enough to lift them to the top of the dispenser all by myself! And the boyfriend? He remained in the picture, happy to be relieved of at least some of my chores.

FIT FOR LIFE

Learning more about strength training has been an inspiring experience. Once I let go of my outdated ideas of what strength training was all about and gave it a try, I quickly realized that I'd found a fitness tool for life.

It's easy to fit into my schedule, there are so many exercises from which to choose, and most important, it makes me feel great!

2 | What Is Strength Training?

BUILDING A BETTER BODY

Once considered an obscure sport practiced mainly by competitive athletes and vain bodybuilders, strength training has become one of the most popular fitness activities in the country, with more than twenty million participants.

Why are so many people including strength training in their fitness routines? Because it works. Improving muscle strength is the best way to build balanced strength throughout the body, giving you the power, stamina, energy, and balance you need to go for long walks, lift a child out of a car seat, carry around a heavy briefcase, or serve a tennis ball with speed and accuracy.

PROGRESSIVE OVERLOAD

Muscles get stronger through a process called *progressive overload*. In your daily life, you lift objects all the time without even thinking about them—the morning newspaper, a pen, a glass of water. You also make movements that require basic strength, such as sitting down and getting up from a chair. If you want to improve muscle strength and functionality, you need to challenge your muscles against *resistance*, or, an amount of weight heavier than they are used to handling.

Strength training exercises are based on such common movements as lifting, pulling, pushing, and squatting. By adding resistance—in the form of weights or in some exercises, your own body weight—to these simple movements and repeating them a specific number of times, you overload your muscles. With regular practice, and by progressively increasing the resistance, muscles gradually adapt to each new load and become stronger.

How Strength Training Affects Muscles

Skeletal muscles are composed of bundles of muscle fibers, blood vessels, nerves, and connective tissue. Because the term *building muscle* is commonly used in the fitness world, people often mistakenly believe that strength training literally builds muscles. Though strength training will not cause new muscles to grow, it does enlarge individual muscle fibers, thereby improving muscle size, shape, endurance, and strength.

Improving Communication and Coordination

As muscle fibers expand, accommodating greater workloads, the blood vessels and nerves serving muscles become more efficient at their jobs. Blood flow increases, bringing more oxygen to muscles, and the nervous system becomes more adept at telling muscles how to work.

For example, when you want to lift a weight or perform a lunge, first your brain has to send a message to your muscles, via nerves, telling them what to do. If these movements are new to you (or if you're adding resistance to them by holding weights), you might feel awkward and have trouble maintaining your balance. With regular practice, the connection between brain and muscles, called a *neuromuscular pathway*, becomes more established, helping you develop coordination as you develop stronger muscles. In other words, as you train your muscles to take on new challenges, you're also training the nerves that connect muscles and brain to carry messages more effectively.

In fact, the initial phase of strength training is really about helping the body adapt to new stresses. During the first four to six weeks of training, people often feel stronger—a powerful motivator for continuing their fitness programs. In reality, they haven't increased the size of their muscles or significantly improved strength, but they've trained the neuromuscular system (i.e., the muscle and nerves) to work more effectively. As the nervous system gets better at recruiting the right muscles for each task and reactivating underused or weak muscles, coordination and balance also improve. With a more stable body and improved skill in performing the exercises, strength training begins to impact muscle size and strength.

Strength Without Bulk

How big your muscles get depends on genetics, gender, and the type of training you do. For example, a very thin person is unlikely to develop hulking muscles from a basic strength training program. Likewise, someone with a heavyset build might increase muscle strength but will need to lose weight before he sees muscle definition. Even people with the same build won't respond to training the same way. The important thing to remember is that all body types can benefit from strength training.

Many women avoid strength training, particularly lifting weights, for fear of developing bulky muscles. The truth is, women don't have the genetic makeup, or the testosterone, to bulk up. Most men won't develop huge muscles from lifting weights either, because basic strength training programs are designed to help improve muscle strength and endurance, not pump up muscles.

It's helpful to keep in mind that strength training is not the same as bodybuilding, an activity designed to create hyper-defined muscles for the sake of achieving a physical aesthetic that is neither natural nor functional. Bodybuilders achieve their chiseled physiques through a specific type of intense training with very heavy weights (and for some, the use of steroids). The training methods in this book are different; they are designed to help you achieve an overall body strength that translates to all of your daily movements and activities.

Types of Strength Training

In the past, strength training was primarily about lifting weights. The "no pain, no gain" motto permeated the gym atmosphere, and "pumping iron" seemed to be more about vanity than health and fitness. If you didn't like lifting weights or were intimidated by the hype, you missed out on the benefits of developing a stronger body.

Today, there's greater awareness of strength training's many benefits and of the many types of strength training exercises. Whether you call it strength training, resistance training, weight training, or weight lifting, it's all about improving muscle strength. With increased options, more people of all ages and fitness levels can feel comfortable starting and maintaining a strength training routine.

Here are a few of the most common strength training modalities:

- *Body weight as resistance.* Many people don't know that it's possible to achieve the benefits of lifting weights without lifting weights. Such exercises as push-ups, back extensions, squats, and lunges—in which you use your body weight as resistance—build muscle strength, duplicating the actions of free weight and machine exercises. Because no equipment is required and these exercises can be done anywhere, they are the most accessible form of resistance training.

- *Free weights.* Lifting weights, specifically dumbbells and barbells *(see Figures 2.1 and 2.2)*, is an excellent way to build strength and improve balance and coordination. During free weight exercises, you lift dumbbells or barbells while sitting, standing, or lying down. To gain the most benefits from these exercises, you have to maintain your posture, use correct form, and move your joints through a full range of motion.

  As a result, this type of training improves strength not only in targeted muscles, but also in postural and other supporting muscles. So, you may be lifting weights to

Figure 2.1 Barbell

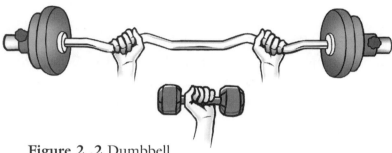

Figure 2 .2 Dumbbell

strengthen your arms or legs, but your abdominal and back muscles get a workout, too. Many fitness experts prefer this training method because the exercises translate directly to real-life movements.

Dumbbells are considered even more effective than barbells because they help you isolate and train each side of the body to equalize strength deficiencies. With barbells, it's possible for your stronger side to compensate for your weaker side. Free weights are ideal home exercise equipment because they are compact and relatively inexpensive.

- *Weight Machines.* Weight machines are ideal for beginners, older adults, and people rehabilitating from illness or injury because they provide support for the body (most exercises are performed while seated or lying on a padded bench), are simple to use, and isolate specific muscles. Using correct form is simpler because you don't have to support your body weight or maintain your balance and the machine determines the range of movement.

   For variety's sake, fitness professionals recommend using a combination of free weights and weight machines for improving strength.

   There are many different types of weight machines that use a variety of resistance methods. Most health clubs have machines that use adjustable stacks of iron weights for resistance. A complete workout involves six to eight machines, however many people don't have the space or the budget to purchase them. The best place to use weight machines is at an accredited health club, gym, YMCA, or YWCA, where a trained professional can instruct you on use. Because this type of instruction is usually part of a health club membership, weight machine exercises won't be covered in this book so that we can focus on exercises you can do at home.

THE BEST APPROACH

You may be wondering which type of strength training is the best. The answer is . . . whichever one works for you. Some people enjoy visiting health clubs or gyms; others prefer exercising at home or at least having the option of doing a few workouts at home every week. Fitness experts may not always agree on the "best" approach, but they do universally recommend selecting a variety of exercises to keep you interested and your muscles challenged.

The workouts in this book, which you'll find in Chapters 9 through 11, were designed with variety, accessibility, and effectiveness in mind. The first workout is a "back to the basics" routine based on common exercises like push-ups and squats that use body weight as resistance. The second workout includes a few weight-free moves and several dumbbell exercises to increase resistance and further challenge balance and coordination. Finally, in Chapter 11, you'll learn a few power moves—combination exercises that challenge upper and lower body at the same time. All of these exercises are relatively simple to learn, yet challenging enough to build real strength. Work-outs can be done at home, at the gym, or anywhere you have a few feet of space.

3 | Benefits of Strength Training

STRENGTH FOR FITNESS AND HEALTH

It's no wonder strength training has become one of the most popular fitness activities in the country. For an exercise that doesn't require a significant time commitment, strength training can produce big results—like making everyday tasks easier, improving your energy, and helping you maintain your weight, prevent injuries, fight disease, and even reverse the effects of aging.

STRENGTH + ENERGY = AN ACTIVE LIFE

Most of us take for granted simple activities like standing in line at the store, sitting at a desk all day, gardening for an afternoon, or enjoying weekend recreational pursuits. At the same time, by middle age, and even as young as thirty, many people begin to feel their age in their backs and joints—not to mention the challenge of maintaining correct posture. Unfortunately, too many people simply accept stiffness, mild pain, and misalignment as part of aging because they don't know that pain isn't normal.

The good news is—getting stronger can help you feel better and stay active. Consistent strength training:

- Improves muscle strength and flexibility throughout the body, restoring function, as well as boosting energy and stamina.
- Restores natural alignment by correcting muscle imbalances and strength deficiencies that contribute to pain, stiffness, and poor posture.
- Promotes joint health by improving flexibility and range of motion and by strengthening the muscles and tissues (i.e., ligaments and tendons) that stabilize them.
- Helps prevent repetitive use and recreational injuries.

GET FIT WITH WEIGHTS

Resistance training isn't just for competitive athletes anymore. Everyone can benefit from improved strength, power, endurance, balance, and coordination.

For people new to exercise, strength training is the first step in becoming more active. Adults of all ages should prepare their bodies for aerobic activities like walking or jogging by first improving muscle strength.

Regular exercisers who include strength training in their routines get more from their workouts. Studies have shown that supplementing aerobic exercise with regular strength training improves strength, endurance, and cardiorespiratory fitness.[1] With greater strength and stamina, you can walk, run, swim, or bike farther before becoming fatigued. And if you're an athlete, you can use strength training to help you throw farther, jump higher, and run faster than your opponents, as well as protect your body from the rigors of strenuous training.

BOOST YOUR MOOD

In addition to pumping up your workouts, resistance training can boost your mood. According to recent studies, intense exercise, including strength training exercises, can produce endorphins—brain chemicals that produce a feeling of well-being—that can last beyond the length of a workout.[2]

Even strength training at moderate intensity can improve your mood by helping you refocus your thoughts and energy. Lifting weights is a wonderful confidence booster. You literally feel stronger as soon as you finish your workout. And with time, as your posture improves and your appearance changes, you'll continue to feel good about yourself.

Participating in a regular strength training program can also combat depression. A Harvard Medical School study showed that 75 percent of clinically depressed men and women who followed a twenty-week strength training program noticed a significant improvement in symptoms.[3]

LIFT WEIGHTS TO LOSE WEIGHT

Being overweight is a risk factor for such life-threatening health problems as diabetes, heart disease, and cancer. With obesity rates reaching epidemic proportions, losing weight and maintaining a healthy weight have never been more important.

The key factor to weight control is maintaining the balance between how many calories you consume and how many you expend. The bottom line is, if you want to prevent weight gain, you have to be active enough to burn off the calories you consume. If you want to lose weight, you have to burn off *more* calories than you consume. Researchers have found that oftentimes people who are overweight aren't eating too much, they're not exercising enough.[4] For those people, simply increasing their activity levels can help control their weight. Others may need a combination of exercise and dietary modifications to lose weight.

Strength training helps you lose or maintain weight by boosting your metabolism in three ways: You burn calories during your workout; you continue to burn calories for a few hours after your workout; and, by increasing your muscle mass, you increase your *resting metabolic rate* so that your body continues to burn calories throughout the day, even when you're not active.

Here's how it works: Muscle tissue burns calories, so as you increase your muscle mass, you'll increase your body's calorie-burning capacity. It's as if your muscles are furnaces that become more efficient at burning fuel. When you think that one pound of muscle burns an average of 45 calories a day, adding just two pounds of muscle through strength training helps you burn 90 more calories each day. That's 630 calories a week, which puts you on track to lose ten pounds in a year.[5]

And here's another weight loss bonus: Studies have shown that dieting alone, or in combination with aerobic exercise, can cause muscle loss along with any fat loss that occurs. Adding strength training to the mix helps dieters maintain and improve muscle mass and strength.

IMPROVE HEART HEALTH

The cardiovascular benefits of aerobic exercise are well known, but many people aren't aware that strength training provides some of the same benefits. Studies have shown that strength training may lower blood pressure, improve heart rate, reduce cholesterol levels (lower LDL or "bad" cholesterol, and increase HDL, "good" cholesterol), and help the heart and lungs work more efficiently—especially when done in combination with aerobic exercise.[6-8]

In the past, strength training was considered too strenuous for people with heart disease. Today, researchers and doctors agree that both aerobic exercise and strength training, when appropriately applied, can be beneficial for some heart patients.[9] In addition to improving heart health, having a stronger body means less strain on the heart during movement (and lifting).

STRONG MUSCLES, STRONG BONES

Osteoporosis, a disease characterized by thinning bones, affects ten million Americans—eight million women and two million men. Another thirty-two million people have osteopenia—low bone mass. Osteoporosis is a serious, but preventable, disease that leaves bones weak and brittle, highly prone to fractures from otherwise harmless falls or movements. Women as young as thirty can get osteoporosis, but postmenopausal women are especially at risk because the onset of menopause causes a natural drop in estrogen, a hormone important to bone health. Without estrogen, bone loss occurs. It's estimated that one out of two women over fifty has osteoporosis.[10]

Both muscle and bone tissue begin to break down beginning at around age thirty to thirty-five as part of the natural aging process. If nothing is done to prevent this deterioration, individuals can lose up to five pounds of muscle in a decade. Women over thirty-five lose 1 percent of their bone mass each year.

Walking is one of the most common forms of exercise, but many women are not aware that it is not enough to prevent osteoporosis. Researchers have found that strength training, as well as weight-bearing aerobic activity, is a key element in building and preserving bone density. Studies have shown that increasing muscle mass helps maintain and improve bone density.[11] To get the most from their fitness programs, walkers should add two or three strength training sessions each week. The more exercise you do before the age of thirty, when the skeletal system is still developing, the better. But if you're over thirty and you've led a sedentary life, it's not too late to start exercising.

ADDITIONAL HEALTH BENEFITS

In addition to protecting heart and bone health, strength training helps fight common diseases such as diabetes and arthritis. Strength training is also used by physical therapists to help people regain functioning after an injury, surgery, or long-term illness.

Studies have shown that:

- Strength training can help prevent the onset of diabetes by reducing body fat, a major risk factor. In addition, increasing muscle mass improves the process by which glucose is used in the body, helping prevent or improve diabetes.[12]
- Strength training may help people with osteoarthritis reduce pain and improve range of motion.[13]
- Strength training may help people with rheumatoid arthritis reduce pain and improve strength.[14]

Reverse the Aging Process

Both improving and maintaining muscle strength become increasingly important as you age. Research confirms that seniors who strength-train can reap the same health, fitness, and emotional benefits as adults forty to sixty years old. Even seniors in their nineties can make strength gains directly related to their quality of life.

Resistance training improves strength, balance, and coordination, which in turn helps prevent falls (and the resulting fractures). Older adults who improve their strength have an easier time getting in and out of bed, going to the bathroom unassisted, and participating in other daily activities. The ability to take care of basic needs is critical for independent living.

Maintaining correct posture is another good reason for seniors to take up weights. Improving overall body strength helps older adults move more efficiently and gracefully, enhancing their appearance and preventing injuries. Greater strength can also help prevent neck pain and a humped upper back ("dowager's hump"), two common postural problems associated with aging.[15]

STRENGTH TRAINING FOR YOU

People strength-train for a variety of reasons. Whatever your reason—and whatever your age, health status, or fitness goals—strength training can help you achieve a stronger, more functional body that's better able to handle all of the demands placed on it.

4 | A Fresh Look at Strength Training

OVERCOMING OBSTACLES

If you're like most people new to strength training, you probably have at least a few questions about how it works and what types of results you can expect from your efforts. Dispelling misconceptions that might be holding you back is the first step to getting started.

Q & A: COMMON MISCONCEPTIONS ABOUT STRENGTH TRAINING

The following questions and answers will help you gain a bit more clarity about what strength training can (and can't) do for you.

Q: Do I have to be strong to strength-train?

A: You don't have to be strong to start a strength training program. In fact, research has shown that beginners can make significant strength gains in a relatively short period of time. Where you begin is based on which exercises challenge your muscles in a way that's appropriate for you. If that's a one-pound weight, or no weight at all, that's okay. As your strength improves, you'll be able to progress to more challenging exercises.

Q: Do I have to spend a lot of time at the gym to gain benefits?

A: You don't have to make a big time commitment or join a health club. Working out at home two or three times a week for twenty to thirty minutes is all you need to do to improve your strength.

Q: Will strength training get rid of my love handles and give me thinner thighs?

A: Strength training, in combination with aerobic exercise and a healthy diet, will help you lose or maintain weight, but it is impossible to "spot reduce," or target a specific area of the body for fat loss. With regular and consistent training your muscles will feel firmer, and you may begin to see improved muscle definition. However, some people may not be able to see much definition until they lose enough weight to reduce the layers of fat covering muscles.

Q: Will lifting weights help me burn more fat?

A: The short answer is yes. The long answer is: The best way to think about fat burning is to focus on total calories burned in any given activity. When you expend calories, some of those calories come from fat and some from carbohydrate. The percentages of fat and carbohydrate burned depends on the activity and on the intensity with which it's performed. For example, walking burns a higher percentage of fat calories than running does, but because running burns so many more total calories, you end up burning more fat calories running than you would in the same amount of time walking. As a "fat burning" exercise, weight lifting falls somewhere between walking and running, with the added benefit of improving *resting metabolic rate* (the ability of the body to continue burning calories for a period of time after you finish exercising).

Q: If I stop working out, will my muscles turn to fat?

A: Fat and muscle are two different tissues. If you stop exercising, you'll lose the strength gains you've made, your muscles will become smaller, and your body will burn fewer calories, but muscle tissue will never turn into fat tissue. If you are deconditioned and want to start strength training again, simply start off where you did as a beginner, gradually progressing to more challenging workouts.

Q: Will lifting weights make me gain weight?

A: Because muscle tissue is denser than fat, you may gain one or two pounds as you increase muscle mass—even if you're slimmer and wearing smaller-size clothing. Don't worry, the added muscle helps you burn more calories, and most people don't train intensely enough to gain significant amounts of weight due to increased muscle mass.

Q: Will strength training make me less flexible?

A: Inactivity, overuse, and strength imbalances are common causes of tight muscles. Strength training challenges muscles through a full range of motion, which increases flexibility. Beginning and following strength training workouts with stretching exercises also helps maintain and improve flexibility.

Q: Will strength training hurt my back (or my knees)?

A: Performed correctly, strength training exercises are safe for healthy people. If you increase your strength, especially in core muscles, you will improve your posture, allowing you to move more efficiently and helping you improve joint strength, thereby reducing the risk of back and joint injuries. If you already have back or knee pain, consult a doctor before beginning a strength training program.

Q: Do I need to eat more protein-rich foods to build muscle?

A: Only exercise will improve muscle strength and size. Most Americans eat plenty of protein, so it's probably not necessary to increase your protein intake unless you're training at a very high level. It is important, though, to eat a healthy, nutritious diet. Including a bit of protein with each meal will help you maintain your energy levels throughout the day.

Q: Do I need to do lower body work if my legs feel strong from running or hiking?

A: Participating in regular aerobic activity is important for cardiovascular health, but it does not build muscle strength or power. Strength training will build balanced strength in your legs and throughout the body, helping you prevent overuse injuries common in repetitive aerobic activities like running.

Q: Can I replace one of my weekly weight workouts with yoga or Pilates?

A: Don't be fooled when you see all the celebrities whose perfect bodies are attributed to yoga or Pilates. Most of those chiseled bodies are the result of frequent and intense activity that most likely includes some strength training.

Yoga and Pilates are both excellent health practices that improve strength, flexibility, balance, and coordination. Some classes can actually be very challenging and leave you with sore muscles. However, most practices will not result in the same strength gains you will make from following a strength training program.

Instead of replacing one workout with another, warm up for your strength training workout with twenty minutes of yoga. Or, if you're strength-training more than twice a week, you could substitute a Pilates or yoga practice for a light strength training workout if the practice addresses all of the major muscle groups.

Q: Can I combine strength training and walking by wearing or carrying weights?

A Fresh Look at Strength Training

A: It's common to see walkers who are wearing ankle or wrist weights. While their intentions are good, the practice is not. Wearing weights will make you work harder, increasing the cardiovascular challenge, but you won't necessarily build muscle strength, because the activity is still primarily an aerobic exercise that builds endurance. Also, wearing weights can place strain on the joints, increasing the risk of injury.

True strength training is based on repetitive exercises with heavier weights than you could carry (and still maintain correct posture) during a walk.

Q: Why does my friend have better muscle definition that I do when I work out harder?

A: Unfortunately, your results are ultimately determined by genetics and body type. There are three main body types: ectomorphs (thin build), mesomorphs (medium build), and endomorphs (heavier build). Some people are predominantly one type, others a combination of types. Each type responds differently to training.

Ectomorphs, who have low amounts of fat and muscle

cells, won't develop huge muscles as they get stronger, but may show definition easily because they don't have much body fat covering their muscles. Mesomorphs, characterized by lower than average fat cells but higher than average muscle cells, will build muscle faster than ectomorphs, and their muscles will look bigger. Endomorphs have higher than average fat cells, but lower than average muscle cells. They will make strength gains, but need to lose weight in order to see a visible change in muscle definition or size.[1]

5 | Meet Your Muscles

BASIC ANATOMY

Before selecting which exercises you want to do, you need to know which muscles to exercise, where they're located, and how they function. Understanding basic anatomy and physiology will improve your ability to visualize your muscles at work, creating a greater mind–body awareness that will help you train more effectively.

Figure 5.1 Muscle Map

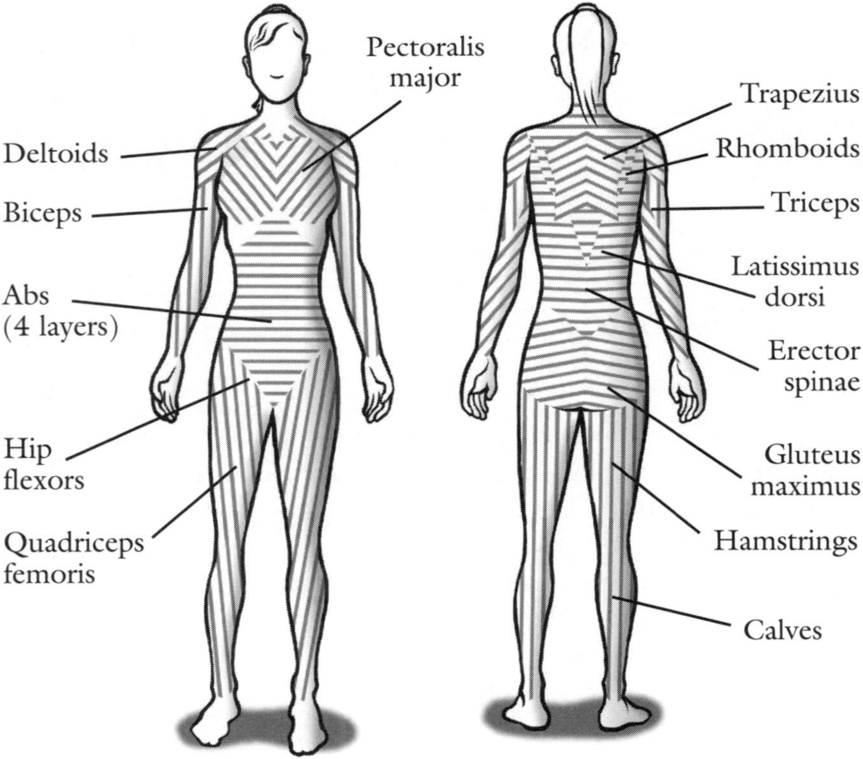

Pectoralis major

Deltoids

Biceps

Abs (4 layers)

Hip flexors

Quadriceps femoris

Trapezius

Rhomboids

Triceps

Latissimus dorsi

Erector spinae

Gluteus maximus

Hamstrings

Calves

Major Muscle Groups

There are more than six hundred muscles in the human body—but you don't have to know them all in order to succeed at strength training. You only need to know the six major muscle groups: located in the back (lower, middle, and upper), chest, shoulders, arms, legs (lower, upper, hips, and buttocks), and abdomen. *(See Figure 5.1.)* These muscles support and stabilize the skeletal system and give your body its shape. The Major Muscle Groups chart on pages 44–45 describes the major muscle groups and their primary functions, and identifies several muscles within each group.[1]

Single- and Multi-Joint Movements

In addition to having a basic understanding of muscle location and function, it's helpful to remember that muscle groups work together to support the body and to make everyday movements. Strength training is based on two types of movements that strengthen both muscles in opposing pairs and several muscles involved in a chain of movement.

Single-joint movements (also called isolation exercises) involve only one joint. For example, your biceps bend your arm; your triceps straighten it. Multi-joint movements (also called compound exercises) involve more than one joint and call into play large muscles (like the quadriceps, hamstrings, and hips that support the weight of the body) and smaller supporting muscles (like the calves and arms). For example, when you want to pick up a bag of groceries, you first have to lower your body to the floor by bending your knees, then pull the object close to you with your arms, and then return to a standing position. The chain of movement involves muscles in your legs, feet, torso, arms, and hands, as well as several joints.

MAJOR MUSCLE GROUPS

Muscle location	Muscle name	Classification	Function
Back	Trapezius	Large muscle	Moves shoulder blade, extends neck, rotates head, and aids in posture.
Back	Latissimus dorsi (called "lats")	Large muscle	Moves shoulder and upper arm, and aids in posture.
Back	Rhomboids	Large muscle	Moves shoulder blade.

Meet Your Muscles

Muscle location	Muscle name	Classification	Function
Back	Erector spinae	Large muscle	Extends back, aids in side bending and rotation of torso and head.
Chest	Pectoralis major (called "pecs")	Large muscle	Moves arm.
Shoulders	Deltoids	Large muscle	Raises arm.
Hips	Hip flexors (including Iliacus, psoas)	Large muscle	Raises leg.
Leg	Quadriceps femoris (called "quads")	Large muscle	Extends knee (to straighten leg).
Leg	Hamstrings	Large muscle	Extends thigh, flexes knee (to bend leg).
Leg	Calves (gastrocnemius and soleus)	Small muscle	Flexes ankle.
Buttocks	Gluteus maximus (called "glutes")	Large muscle	Extends hip, moves pelvis.
Arm	Biceps	Small muscle	Flexes elbow (to bend arm).
Arm	Triceps	Small muscle	Extends elbow (to straighten arm).
Abdomen	Transverse abdominis, internal obliques, external obliques, rectus abdominis	Large muscle	Bends (forward and to the side) and rotates torso.

ELEMENTS OF SUCCESS

A successful strength training routine includes both single- and multi-joint exercises to build balanced strength throughout the body. It should also prepare you for all of the physical demands placed on your body, be part of an overall fitness plan including aerobic and flexibility exercises, and be appropriate for your health and skill level.

6 | Strength Training Guidelines

STRONGER BY DESIGN

As you read in Chapter 2, the key to building stronger muscles is repeatedly overloading them with resistance, then progressively increasing that resistance.

The progressive overload principle is based on several factors, including the amount of resistance used in an exercise (i.e., how heavy the weights are), the number of times the exercise is performed (called "repetitions" or "reps"), and the intensity, duration, and frequency of workouts. How these factors are applied in training determines the efficacy of strengthening exercises.

Fortunately, fitness experts have already determined several general training formulas based on specific goals such as increasing endurance or improving strength. Although there's always room for variations based on individual needs and goals, the following formulas can be used as general guidelines, appropriate for beginning and intermediate level exercisers.

RESISTANCE AND REPS

To improve muscle endurance, fitness experts recommend lifting less than 70 percent of the maximum you can lift, repeating the exercise ten to fifteen (or more) times. If improving strength is your goal, the formula changes, emphasizing heavier weights (between 70 and 80 percent of your max) and fewer reps (8 to 10), lifting until muscles become fatigued.

Many fitness professionals and organizations recommend 8 to 12 reps for strength building. The range in this book is lower to make sure that your exercises build strength. It's easy over time to repeatedly do 12 reps for each exercise, gradually turning your strength workout into more of an endurance workout. To avoid that pitfall, make sure that you lift weights heavy enough to produce fatigue as you approach the highest number in the range.

Figuring out an appropriate resistance level is easier than it sounds. There are no complicated calculations; just select a weight that you can lift at least as many times as the lowest suggested rep (8 for strength building, 10 for endurance), which becomes too heavy to lift while maintaining correct form at the highest rep (10 for strength building, 15 or more for endurance).

Beginners and older adults are encouraged to start with an endurance-focused program (high reps, low weight) and gradually progress to a strength-oriented workout, reducing the number of reps performed by increasing the amount of weight lifted.

These formulas are most easily applied to exercises in which dumbbells, barbells, or weight machines are used. You'll find that when using your own body weight as resistance, as in a push-up or lunge, sometimes you'll only be able to do 4 or 5 reps. That's fine. Other movements may feel much easier, and you'll be able to do more than 10 reps. When this happens, you need to modify those exercises, increasing the difficulty, in order to build strength. (Note: All of the exercises mentioned throughout this book can be found in Chapters 9 to 11.)

SINGLE VS. MULTIPLE SETS

In strength training, reps are organized into groups called *sets*. Each group of repetitions, whether it's 8, 10, 12, 15, or more, makes up a set. Until recently, the common strength training prescription was 3 sets per exercise. This is still the recommended protocol for athletes and people trying to lose weight or change body composition.

For beginners, research has shown that significant strength gains can be made training with 1 set per exercise. Studies with untrained adults have demonstrated that the extra effort of performing 2 or 3 sets may not be reflected proportionately in greater results.[1] However, once exercisers progress past the initial training stage, which usually lasts from three to six months, they need to add more sets, increase resistance, and/or train more frequently to continue making strength gains.[2]

Maintaining Intensity and Interest

Maintaining an appropriate intensity level is an important part of successful training. Intensity refers to how hard you work to perform each strengthening exercise and each complete routine. Many people, especially women, make the common mistake of not training hard enough. Others may regularly practice challenging routines, but experience plateaus where their improvement levels off after several months. To stay motivated and continue making progress, fitness experts recommend varying your workouts every four to six weeks.

Here are several simple ways to maintain your intensity and interest:[3]

- *Mix it up.* If you usually begin your workout with upper body exercises, start with lower body exercises.

- *Exercise more frequently.* If you usually work out twice a week, add one or more workouts a week.

- *Add more reps or sets.* If you've been doing 1-set workouts, try adding 1 or 2 more sets of each exercise. Or, if you've only been doing 8 reps for each exercise, try doing 10.

- *Increase resistance.* Gradually increase the weights you're using by two to three pounds, as long as you can do so without sacrificing form. If you're using body weight as resistance, vary the exercise to make it more challenging. For example, change the hand position in a push-up or hold dumbbells while performing a lunge.

- *Try new exercises.* If you've been doing push-ups for upper body strength, switch to chest press with dumbbells and triceps kickbacks. If you've been using free weights, try weight machines.

- *Pick up the pace.* Take shorter rest breaks between sets.

When incorporating changes, please remember to increase your workload gradually. You don't want to overwhelm yourself or risk injury by changing more than one variable at a time. Even small adjustments can make a difference.

NUMBER, TYPE, AND ORDER OF EXERCISES

A basic strength training program should contain between seven and ten exercises, performed in a specific order, that work all of the major muscle groups.

The following information, adapted from the National Strength and Conditioning Association, will help you organize your workouts.[4] As you practice the workouts in Chapters 9 through 11, you'll notice that they were designed according to these six guidelines.

1. *Work large muscles first.* It doesn't matter if you train your upper or lower body first, but you should train large muscles (chest, back, shoulders, thighs, and hips) before you address smaller muscles (lower legs and arms).

    Large muscles, primarily responsible for movement and posture, are your strongest muscles, able to handle the stress of training, while smaller, secondary muscles are designed to support primary muscles. If you train them first, they can become too fatigued to do their jobs.

    Since you'll be using your abdominal muscles in all of the exercises, add abs exercises in the middle or end of your workout to prevent fatiguing them too much before you finish your workout.

2. *Start with and focus on multi-joint exercises.* To build balanced, integrated strength throughout the body, your training should predominantly be based on compound movements, exercises like the push-up and squat, which involve two or more joints. Practicing multi-joint exercises helps strengthen both large and small muscles and connective tissues, promoting balance, coordination, and joint stability. Within a workout, do your multi-joint moves for each body part before single-joint exercises. For example, perform push-ups, shoulder press, or other compound upper body movements before the biceps curl and the triceps overhead extension.

3. *Alternate pushing and pulling movements.* Again, for balanced strength and joint stability, you need to train muscles that perform opposite actions in the body. Make sure that your workout includes pushing exercises such as the chest press or push-up and pulling exercises like the one-arm row or pull-up. This applies to your legs, too. For instance, the

squat predominantly works your quadriceps, duplicating a pushing movement. The lunge, which emphasizes the hamstrings more, is considered a "pulling" movement.

4. *Train one body part at a time.* Complete all of the exercises for each body part before moving on to the next muscle group. For example, do all of your chest exercises before you move on to your shoulder exercises. Also, in exercises that work one side of the body at a time, remember to perform the same number of reps and sets on each side of the body.

5. *Train complementary muscles.* Complementary muscles are muscles that work together in a chain of movement so that you can perform tasks like throwing a ball or lifting a glass from the table to your mouth. If you follow the previous instructions (basing your workouts on multi-joint exercises) you'll be including exercises that work such complementary muscle pairs as the back and biceps (one-arm row) and the chest and triceps (push-up).

6. *Vary your approach.* You can alternate upper and lower body exercises throughout a workout to give your muscles more

recovery time or perform all upper body exercises before lower body exercises (or vice versa) to increase the intensity in each major muscle group.

FREQUENCY AND DURATION

One of the best things about strength training is that you don't have to do it every day. In fact, strength training on consecutive days is not recommended, unless you alternate working the lower body one day and the upper body the next day. For best results, you need to allow forty-eight hours of recovery time between each workout.

You do need to strength-train at least twice a week, however, to make strength gains. Strength training workouts can be very efficient, though, and in the time it takes to watch your favorite sitcom, you can complete seven to ten exercises. Allow twenty to forty minutes for each workout; your time will vary depending on how many sets you perform and how long you rest between sets.

Strength Training Guidelines

Training goal	Resistance	Reps	Sets	Frequency (times per week)
Muscle endurance	<70% of max	10–15 (or more)	2–3	2–3 (on nonconsecutive days)
Muscle strength	70–80%+ of max	8–10	1–3	2–3 (on nonconsecutive days)

REST AND RECOVERY

To maintain intensity, move through your workouts at a steady pace. This will become easier to do as you become more proficient in performing each exercise. Ideally, rest for thirty seconds between sets. Initially, you may need to take sixty- to ninety-second rest breaks. Of course, if you feel overly tired or dizzy, rest for a longer period. If you feel pain or your dizziness persists, stop exercising.

Try not to overdo it by performing too many reps or by lifting weights that are too heavy for you. It's common to experience muscle soreness during the initial stages of a strength training program as your body adapts to the demands of exercise. It is safe to train with mild soreness, but if your muscle soreness persists for more than forty-eight hours, wait an extra day before your next workout. If you continue to experience muscle soreness, it could be a sign that you're training too hard, not practicing exercises in correct form, or using weights that are too heavy for you.

7 | Techniques for Successful Strength Training

EFFICIENT, EFFECTIVE WORKOUTS

The key to successful strength training is using correct form. Knowing how to prepare for and safely execute every move will help you get the most from your workouts.

STAND UP STRAIGHT

Your body is strongest and most able to perform such tasks as squatting to work in the garden, walking to the store, pushing open a heavy door, or lifting weights when it is correctly aligned. Stop for a moment now and practice correct posture, described below:

> Stand tall with feet hips-width apart and firmly planted on the floor, legs straight with knees slightly bent, abs gently engaged to keep pelvis and lower back in their neutral positions, back straight, chest slightly lifted, arms hanging at sides, shoulders relaxed and away from ears, neck long, and head resting on top of spine, chin parallel to floor, and eyes looking straight ahead. In this position, your ankles, knees, hips, shoulders, and ears all line up with each other.

Do you notice that standing up straight is actually more relaxing than standing all hunched over? Or that you can breathe easier? Memorize what it feels like to stand tall without being rigid. Maintaining this alignment in all of your daily activities will help your body function more efficiently.

[Note: As you can see in Figure 7.1, a straight back doesn't mean a flat back. The back has three natural curves—a slight inward curve at the lower back (lumbar curve), a slight outward curve at mid-back (thoracic curve), and a slight inward curve at the neck (cervical curve). The goal of correct posture is maintaining the natural alignment of these three curves.]

Neutral Spine

One indicator of correct posture is neutral spine, the position of the spine—particularly, the lower back—in optimal alignment. In other words, it's the spinal position best able to bear the weight of your body. Fitness experts recommend maintaining neutral spine throughout the day, and especially during exercise, to

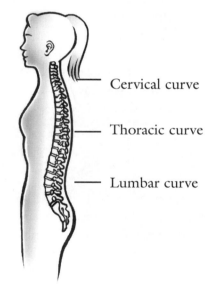

Cervical curve

Thoracic curve

Lumbar curve

Figure 7.1 Spine

protect the lower back and promote good posture. Try this simple exercise to figure out where neutral spine is for you:

> Lie on the floor, with your feet flat on the floor, heels about a foot away from buttocks. Using your abdominal muscles, slowly and gently press your lower back to the floor. Notice how your pelvis rolls backward. Next, using your lower back muscles, slowly and gently arch your lower back, noticing how your pelvis rolls forward. Return to starting position. Neutral spine is the position between arched and flattened.

USE YOUR ABS

Most people don't think about the fact that all movement goes through the torso or that their abdominal muscles are vitally important for posture and spinal support. Part of maintaining correct posture and practicing strength training exercises safely is using the abdominal muscles to facilitate movement and to protect the lower back.

Techniques for Successful Strength Training

There are four layers of abdominal muscles located between your pelvis and rib cage. Along with the back muscles, they form a corset of support for the spine. When performing strength training exercises, always stabilize the spine before making any movements. Contracting your abdominal muscles by pulling them up and in toward your spine (starting with the deepest layer and working up to the most superficial layers) will help you maintain correct posture and neutral spine, protecting your lower back from injury and helping you maintain your balance in moves that challenge your stability. Some fitness instructors call this action "navel to spine."

If you're not sure how to engage these muscles, visualize that you have a zipper deep in your abdomen, beginning at your pubic bone and ending at your sternum. As you zip your abdomen shut, your abdominal muscles act like a corset, pulling tighter around your middle. (For more detailed information about how your abdominal and back muscles function, and about building core strength, consult *The Little Pilates Book* or *The Little Abs Workout Book* from my fitness series.)

Six Lifting Techniques

You'll notice in the workout chapters that most of the instructions relate to your stance, posture, and form. The actual lifting phase takes just a few seconds. Following these six technique tips will help you practice correct form:

1. *Activate Abs.* Once in starting position, pull your abs up and in toward your spine before performing each exercise. By maintaining abs contraction throughout each exercise, you will maintain neutral spine and correct posture, and protect the lower back from injury.

2. *Practice control.* Use slow, controlled movements through a full range of motion to raise and lower weights. Move joints within their natural plane of movement. For instance, when you do a biceps curl, you'll bring the weight to the same side shoulder because that's the way the joint hinges. The same principle applies with the shoulder press: you'll raise the dumbbells until they're aligned over your shoulders.

   As a general rule, take two seconds to lift a weight (or make the initial exertion) and four seconds to lower it back into starting position. The exception to this rule would be squats and lunges, in which you'll take four seconds to lower your body and two to raise it, pausing briefly in between.

3. *Pay attention to form*. In addition to maintaining correct posture, pay attention to the instructions; they describe how body parts should align with each other to maintain a healthy body position in which to work against resistance in dumbbell and weight-free exercises.

4. *Use your head*. Concentrate on correct form and visualize your muscles at work to help you increase body awareness and stay on task.

5. *Stay smooth*. Do not sway your body or use jerky movements, momentum, or gravity to lift or lower weights. If you want to succeed in making true strength changes, you must work your muscles during both the lifting and lowering phases of the exercise. It may sound funny, but try to be graceful, performing each move with intent and progressing smoothly from exercise to exercise.

Caution: Remember to use ergonomic lifting techniques when retrieving and storing weights.

6. *Breathe!* Remember to breathe; holding your breath can be harmful. Instead, use your breath to facilitate movement, exhaling with the lift and inhaling as you return to starting position.

TAKE YOUR TIME

Life can be so hectic; try to resist rushing through your workout to get to your next appointment. Instead, try thinking about exercise as a time to let go of responsibilities, relax, and pay close attention to yourself. Strength training exercises provide you with a great opportunity to know your body better. Viewing your workout as enjoyable and beneficial will help you have more fun and make the time go by faster. Remember to pace yourself, and don't try to progress too quickly.

WARM UP, COOL DOWN

Always warm up before exercising to help reduce your risk of injury. A good warm-up consists of five to ten minutes of low intensity aerobic activity (walking, jogging, or riding a stationary bike) followed by five to ten minutes of stretching, addressing all of the major muscle groups. These activities increase blood flow to the muscles and improve muscle and connective tissue suppleness, preparing the body for exercise.

SIX STRETCHING TIPS[1]

1. Ease yourself into each stretch using slow, controlled movements.
2. You will feel tension in the muscle; do not push beyond that tension.
3. Do not use jerky or bouncing movements.
4. Relax your body and continue breathing, inhaling and exhaling slowly and rhythmically.
5. Hold stretch for about thirty seconds, then slowly release.
6. Stretch all major muscle groups: chest, back, abs, shoulders, arms, and legs.

Cooling down after your workout is equally important. Stretching your muscles after all of the muscle contractions involved in strength training will help you retain your flexibility and range of motion. In fact, studies show that strength and flexibility gains are greater when stretching is added to strength training routines. Some people like to do brief stretches during the rest breaks between sets. That's fine, but you'll still need to include a few minutes of dedicated stretching after your workout. For more information about stretching, check out the many sources available, including books, videos, certified personal trainers, and physical therapists.

STAY HYDRATED

In addition to drinking the recommended eight glasses of water a day for optimal health, keep a bottle of water on hand when exercising. Dehydration can sneak up on you . . . by the time you feel thirsty, you're usually already a bit dehydrated. There's no need to drown yourself, but drinking before, during, and after your workout can help you prevent dehydration.

8 | Getting Started

BEFORE YOU BEGIN

Congratulations! Making the commitment to improve your strength is an excellent way to reap many health and fitness benefits. It's never easy to make changes, and starting a new fitness routine can be daunting. So give yourself credit for taking on this challenge.

By reading to this point in *The Little Strength Training Book*, you've already taken the first step in getting stronger, fitter, and leaner. The next step is learning just a few more tips that will help you prepare physically and mentally for beginning your new strength training workout.

Self-Assessment

Before you begin any exercise program, it's a good idea to assess your health and your fitness level. Think about your lifestyle, your posture, any health concerns you might have, and your current strength. If you're like most people, you probably feel strong in some areas of your body and weaker in others. Or maybe you've noticed that spending most days sitting at a desk or behind the wheel of a car has affected your posture. Spending a few minutes on self-assessment will help you start identifying your training goals.

Talk to Your Doctor

Consult with your physician before beginning any new exercise program, especially if you have a known medical condition. Take this book along and show your doctor which exercises you'd like to do. The workouts are appropriate for many healthy adults, but some of the exercises could be harmful to people with certain health conditions. Even healthy people may need to modify some exercises or even try different exercises.

If you are an older adult, pregnant, or have existing injuries or diseases, your doctor might refer you to a physical therapist who can modify the exercises or prescribe new exercises if necessary.

If your child (age eight or older) is interested in beginning a strength training program, consult his or her physician, then find a strength training program designed and supervised by a fitness professional experienced in youth training techniques.

Ask for Help

Reading this book is a great way to learn more about strength training, but don't be afraid to ask for help if you need it. Especially if you're new to exercise, working with a certified personal trainer, a certified strength and conditioning specialist, or a licensed physical therapist is the best way to learn how to perform all of the exercises correctly. An experienced fitness professional can also personalize the workouts in this book, modifying or adding exercises if necessary.

A session with a trainer generally costs between $30 and $75 an hour. Some trainers will work with two or three people at once at a reduced rate. Learning correct form so that you can exercise safely on your own is well worth the expense of one or two sessions. Another great source of strength training information are strength training classes, now popular at many health clubs.

Setting Goals

A good strength training program should be designed around your fitness goals. Having clear short- and long-term goals will help you select the appropriate exercises, as well as stay focused and motivated. Consider your resources and schedule so that you can decide what type of equipment you want to use, where you want to exercise (home or gym), and how much time you can devote to exercise. Working out with a friend can help you stay on track.

When planning your workouts, set realistic, attainable goals.

For example, trying to lose twenty pounds in three months might not be possible; instead, try losing two to three pounds a month.

What to Expect

The best thing about lifting weights is that you'll feel stronger even after your first workout, and this feeling, along with improved mood and energy, will keep you motivated.

During the first four to six weeks of a new strength training program, the body goes through an adaptation phase where nerves are retrained and muscles reactivated to function more optimally. So even though you'll feel like you're getting stronger, 80 percent of your strength gains will simply be a reflection of becoming more skilled at performing the exercises. Don't be discouraged by this process, though, because this critical period lays the foundation for real strength gains to occur.

After about six weeks, your hard work begins to improve muscle strength and size. During this phase, you'll get stronger, and gradually, you'll start noticing some results. Within two months, you'll feel firmer and more flexible, your balance will

THE LITTLE STRENGTH TRAINING BOOK

improve by 30 to 50 percent, and you'll have more energy and stamina to pursue recreational and athletic pursuits. You'll be able to walk farther and faster, move more quickly and serve more powerfully on the tennis court, lift and carry everyday objects with greater ease, or spend more time gardening before becoming fatigued or sore. As you progress with your training, you'll be able to lift heavier weights and exercise more frequently, further boosting your skills and confidence.

If you want to . . .	Practice these exercises . . .
Banish upper arm flab	Overhead Triceps Extension (or Triceps Kickback), Push-up, Biceps Curl
Prevent dowager's hump	One-Arm Row, Back Extension, Superperson, Pull-up, Bicycle, Vertical Crunch
Tone your thighs	Squat, Lunge, One-Legged Squat
Flatten your stomach	Vertical Crunch, Bicycle

Getting Started

If you want to . . .	Practice these exercises . . .
Strengthen your back	Back Extension, Superperson, One-Arm Row, Pull-up
Improve your balance	Squat, Lunge, One-Legged Squat
Shape your shoulders	Shoulder Press, Push-up
Steel your buns	Squat, Lunge, One-Legged Squat
Firm up your pecs	Push-up, Dumbbell Press (or Dumbbell Fly)

*For detailed instructions see Chapters 9 and 10.

Results

In a study of untrained adults, where subjects participated in two or three twenty-five-minute weekly weight-lifting sessions (using weight machines) over an eight- to twelve-week period, women gained an average of two pounds of muscle, lost four pounds of fat, and improved strength by 40 percent. Men gained an average of four pounds of muscle, lost seven pounds of fat, and improved strength by 55 percent.[1]

Of course, results will vary from person to person. Changes in appearance or strength are determined by how frequently and how intensely you train, your body type, and other factors like diet and gender. People trying to lose a significant amount of weight should allow four to six months for changes in appearance.

TENSION VS. PAIN

Strength training is very safe if you follow the guidelines, pay attention to your form, and don't try lifting more than you can handle. If you're new to exercise, it might take you some time to understand the significance of the different sensations you'll feel in your muscles.

You may feel tension and a slight burning sensation in your working muscles when you perform strength training exercises, but you should never feel sharp, sudden, or stabbing pain in any part of the body. If you start with light weights and gradually increase, you'll get a sense of what your muscles feel like when they're working. You want to challenge them, not strain them.

If at any time you feel dizzy, lightheaded, or experience a sharp or stabbing pain in your knees, back, or other part of the body, slowly lower the weight until you can put it down safely on a raised surface or the floor, using your legs to lower your body and holding the weight close to your body. Then sit or lie down. If the dizziness or pain does not stop, get help immediately.

YOUR FITNESS PLAN

So whose exercise guidelines do you follow when one organization recommends thirty minutes of exercise a day and another recommends sixty? It depends on your fitness and health goals.

First, it's important to note that there's a difference between gaining health benefits and achieving optimal strength and functioning. The exercise guidelines prescribed by such organizations as the American College of Sports Medicine or the U.S.

Surgeon General refer to the amount, intensity, and frequency of exercise that can impart health benefits. Of course, these guidelines can be adapted to suit individual needs, limitations, and training goals. For instance, inexperienced exercisers or older adults may be advised by their doctors, physical therapists, or personal trainers to begin with less than the recommended amount of exercise and gradually work up to more activity. For some people thirty minutes a day might be adequate.

The recent sixty-minute recommendation made by the Institute of Medicine's Food and Nutrition Board and endorsed by the American Council on Exercise was suggested with our national obesity epidemic in mind and was based on an amount of activity that has been shown in research studies to help people maintain a healthy weight and cardiovascular health. So, if you're trying to lose weight, change your body shape, or improve athletic performance, you may need to do more than some guidelines recommend in order to reach your goals.

As a general rule, strength training is most effective when it's part of an overall fitness plan that includes regular aerobic exercise and a healthy diet. The American College of Sports Medicine, regarded by fitness professionals as one of the top resources for health and fitness information, recommends the following exercise prescription for developing cardiovascular fitness, muscle strength, and flexibility:[2]

- Twenty to sixty minutes of *moderate intensity* physical activity three to five days a week. (Moderate intensity means that you're working hard enough to work up a sweat, but not too hard to carry on a conversation with a workout partner. Physical activity can be cumulative throughout the day. For example, running or brisk walking twice a day for fifteen minutes equals one thirty-minute period of exercise.)
- Physical activity should involve large muscle groups, such as those used in walking, jogging, climbing stairs, swimming, shoveling snow, and cycling.
- Strength training two to three days a week, performing a minimum of one set of 8–12 reps of 8–10 exercises.
- Stretching major muscle groups two to three days a week.

APPAREL AND EQUIPMENT

You don't need to wear anything special for strength training, just comfortable clothes that allow you to move freely. Some people prefer loose clothing, like sweats or shorts and a T-shirt, others like more form-fitting tanks and shorts. Always wear athletic shoes to keep your feet safe. Your shoes should have good support, nonslip soles, and control foot motion during side-to-side movements.

As for equipment . . . all you need are dumbbells, sold at most sporting goods stores for between $6 and $20 per set, depending on the brand and style. Molded dumbbells come in many styles, including chrome, hexagonal shaped, vinyl coated, and neoprene coated, with wide and narrow hand grips. You can also buy dumbbell bars and plates so that you can adjust the dumbbells as you progress. Whichever style you prefer, don't buy the first set you see; look around and try out a few to find the weights that you like best. Garage sales are a great place to find inexpensive (and often only lightly used) weights.

You'll need two or three different sets of dumbbells since you'll be able to lift more weight in some exercises than in others. For women, teens, and older adults, a set of 3-pound, 5-pound, and 8-pound dumbbells makes a great starter set (men may need to start with 8-pound, 10-pound, and 12-pound weights). As you progress, you can buy more dumbbells (or trade with friends). In the back of the book, you'll find a list of several companies that sell a variety of strength training equipment.

WEARING WEIGHTS

As stated previously, wearing ankle or wrist weights is not an effective way to improve strength, and can strain joints. The best way to wear your weights would be an all-body suit in which the weight could be evenly distributed across the body. Since these suits don't exist (yet), the next best thing is a weighted vest. Many people use weighted vests to increase the intensity of their workouts and as a substitute for dumbbells in exercises like lunges and squats. Expect to pay at least $60 for a quality weighted vest.

EVALUATING PROGRESS

After a few months of strength training, you can evaluate your progress in several ways. First, notice the weights you're using. If they're heavier than the dumbbells you started with, you've made strength gains. Another measure of increased strength is your ability to add more sets to your workout. If you started with one set of each exercise and can move up to two or three sets, that's progress.

If you want visual proof, look in the mirror after a shower and see if your body looks firmer. Losing a few pounds is another indicator that your hard work is producing benefits. You can also measure around your biceps to see if they've increased in size or measure your waist (women should measure around the hips since that's where they store fat) to see if you've lost some weight. Of course, don't expect huge measurements. Changes of one-half to one inch are significant.

STAY FOCUSED, HAVE FUN

As with any fitness endeavor, your progress will be gradual, and you'll need to practice regularly to see results. Be patient with yourself, stay focused on your goals, and by all means, remember that you're doing something that's going to help you look and feel better. Enjoy it!

9 | Back to Basics: The Weight-Free Workout

IMPROVING OVERALL STRENGTH

Practicing weight-free exercises is an effective way to improve overall strength, learn correct form, master strength training techniques, and prepare your body for the next level of strength training: lifting weights.

WEIGHT-FREE EXERCISES

The following weight-free workout was designed to improve overall strength by working the body's major muscle groups through compound, multi-joint movements. This type of training strengthens and improves functioning in the muscles primarily responsible for all of the daily movements our bodies make.

All of the exercises in this workout, and throughout *The Little Strength Training Book*, were selected and reviewed for accuracy and safety under the guidance of two certified athletic trainers and a licensed physical therapist, all of whom are also certified strength and conditioning specialists.

HOW TO PERFORM THE EXERCISES

In each exercise, you'll be using your own body weight as resistance. At first glance, the exercises may appear to be very simple because they are based on common movements. However, once you get down on the floor and try to do your first push-up, you'll soon realize that correctly performing the exercises can be quite challenging.

Don't feel discouraged if you can only do a few of some exercises, like push-ups. The harder you have to work to perform just a few reps means that you're getting a strength workout from that exercise. People who have an easy time lifting their own body weight will need to find ways to make certain exercises more difficult so that they are only able to perform 8–10 reps.

HOW TO FOLLOW THE INSTRUCTIONS

If you haven't already read the first eight chapters of this book, please do so before trying any of the exercises or workouts in this book. Understanding the guiding principles and techniques of strength training will help you train safely and effectively.

When you're ready to begin a workout, read through the complete texts for all of the exercises so that you get a sense of the movements you'll be making and how to coordinate them with your breath. Then, before you begin each exercise, read each individual set of instructions again. Instructions are accompanied by an illustration (or two) depicting the essence of the move. Use the illustration to help you become familiar with each exercise, but please don't neglect to read all of the information provided.

ORDER OF EXERCISES

After a five- to ten-minute warm-up that includes light aerobic activity and stretching all the major muscle groups, perform the exercises in the following order. (*Exception*: If you choose to do the optional pull-up exercise it should be performed after the push-up.)

1. Push-up
2. Back Extension
3. Bicycle
4. Squat
5. Lunge
6. Pull-up (optional)

You'll notice that there are two versions of the lunge exercise. Choose one each time you do this workout. After four to eight weeks, you can change the order, practicing the lower body exercises first, as follows: squat, lunge, push-up, pull-up (optional), back extension, bicycle. You can also work the abs in between the upper and lower body exercises. Follow this workout by stretching all of the major muscle groups again.

CHEST

EXERCISE 1: PUSH-UP

The push-up is a fitness classic, a challenging exercise that effectively strengthens the upper body. If you've ever done push-ups before, you know that they are very difficult. You may only be able to do one or two initially, but don't let that discourage you. With time and practice, you'll be able to do more than you ever imagined. If necessary, try the modified push-up.

Targets: Chest, shoulders, triceps, and abs
Duplicates: Bench Press with free weights or Chest Press on a machine

Starting Position

Kneel on your hands and knees, with your hands lined up underneath your shoulders. Extend your legs, one at a time, until you are balancing on your toes and hands. Your body should be straight, with ankles, knees, hips, shoulders, and ears in line with each other. Keep abs pulled up and in toward spine throughout this exercise to protect your lower back and help you stay in correct form.

Action

1. Bend your arms, lowering your chest to the floor. You don't have to touch your chest to the floor, but try to get within 2–4 inches.

2. Push against the floor with your hands, raising your body back into starting position. Do as many reps as you can.

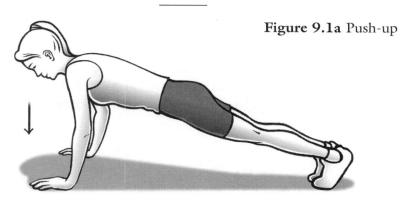

Figure 9.1a Push-up

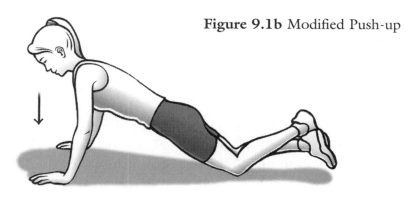

Figure 9.1b Modified Push-up

Technique Tips

- Keep legs together, body straight.
- Inhale as you lower your body, exhale as you raise it.
- Do not lock your arms in the extended position.

Modifications

- From the raised starting position, you can lower your knees to the ground, keeping feet in the air (a few inches above the floor), ankles crossed. *(See Figure 9.1b.)*
- You can also do push-ups against a wall or the edge of a countertop.

Progressions

- Make push-ups harder by performing them more slowly. Try to take 2–3 seconds to lower your body, pause for 1–2 seconds in that position, then take 2–3 seconds to raise your body.
- Widen your hand position to focus on your chest, narrow hand position to focus on triceps.

- Try doing push-ups with both hands holding a medicine ball, with one hand at a time, or with one hand raised on an aerobics step.

BACK

EXERCISE 2: BACK EXTENSION

The back is often the most neglected area in strength training because many people mistakenly believe that challenging the back muscles will hurt them. The truth is, you need to strengthen back muscles in order to maintain a healthy back, prevent low back pain, and develop balanced core strength. The back extension is an excellent exercise for strengthening lower back muscles responsible for stabilizing the spine, forward bending of the torso, and posture. Modifying the arm position of this move helps work the trapezius muscle of the mid-back.

Targets: Back (erector spinae), shoulders
Duplicates: Stiff-Legged Dead Lift with barbell or Back Extension on machine

Starting Position

Lie facedown on the floor, with your head turned to the right, arms at sides (palms up), legs together, tops of feet against the floor.

Action

1. Pulling your abs up and in toward the spine, press the front of your hips and pubic bone into the floor and raise your chest 4–8 inches off the floor, keeping your neck straight. As you raise your chest, pull your hands several inches away from torso and rotate your arms so that your palms face down. This movement helps flatten the shoulder blades in the upper back.

2. Pause in this raised position and take 2–4 breaths, inhaling and exhaling slowly and deliberately.

3. Slowly lower your chest to the floor, rotating your arms back to their original positions, and resting the left side of your

Figure 9.2a Back Extension

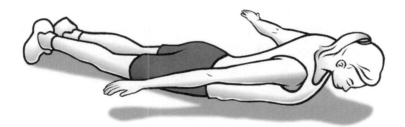

Figure 9.2b Modified Back Extension

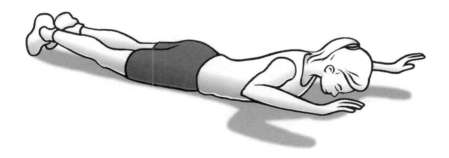

face on the floor. Do 1–3 sets of 8–10 reps. With each rep, alternate resting the right and left sides of your face on the floor when lowering your chest and head to the floor. (Note: Follow this exercise with an effective lower back stretch.)

Technique Tips

- Keep abs pulled up and in toward spine as you raise and lower your upper body. Contracting your glutes (i.e., squeezing together buttocks) will also help protect your back. Keep legs against floor.
- Look at the floor to keep neck straight.

Modification

- To work the muscles of the mid-back, too, begin with your arms bent at 90° so that your arms are parallel, on each side of your head, palms down. Then squeeze together your shoulder blades as you raise your chest off the floor (raise chest and arms as one unit, keeping arms bent). Keep neck straight. *(See Figure 9.2b.)*

Progressions

- Increase the challenge by performing this exercise more slowly, holding the pause for a longer count, and doing more reps or sets.

Caution

- Not recommended for people with osteoporosis. Children and teens who are still growing should not raise their torso past the point of extension, which they'll reach when chest is greater than about 2 inches from the floor.

ABS

EXERCISE 3: BICYCLE

Strong abs are essential for a healthy back. And who doesn't want a flatter, more toned stomach? In a study commissioned by the American Council on Exercise (ACE), researchers rated the bicycle the most effective abs exercise.

Targets: Abs (rectus abdominis, internal and external obliques, and transverse abdominis)

Duplicates: Crunch or Abdominal Curl on a machine

Starting Position

Lie on your back with your knees bent, feet flat on the floor, fingertips placed against the sides of your head, just behind your ears. Pull your abs up and in toward spine. Slowly lift your feet off of the floor, one at a time, and bend knees until they are over your torso. Then raise your upper body until your shoulder blades are no longer touching the floor.

Action

1. Extend your left leg as you bring your left shoulder toward your right knee. Keep your arms wide and in line with your ears. As you bring your left leg back into your body, extend your right leg and bring your right shoulder toward your left knee. Your upper body should remain raised off the floor, abs pulled to spine.

Figure 9.3a Bicycle

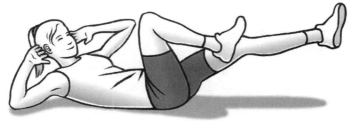

Figure 9.3b Bicycle

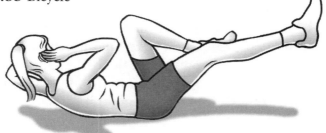

2. Continue alternating legs, as if you're pedaling a bicycle, while simultaneously rotating your torso toward your bent knee. Breathe normally throughout exercise. Do 1 to 3 sets of 8–10 reps.

Technique Tips

- Do not touch your elbows to your knees; the goal is to use the abdominal muscles to rotate the torso. Keeping your arms wide will prevent you from pulling on your head, which can strain the neck, and help you activate the deepest layers of your abdominal muscles.
- Initiate movement from the abs, and lift the chest, shoulders, neck, and head as one unit.
- Although some fitness experts recommend keeping your lower back pressed to the floor during this exercise to protect the lower back, it's best to maintain neutral spine if you can. Beginners, or those with weak abs, might want to keep their backs pressed to the floor until they have developed the abdominal strength to maintain neutral spine.

Modification

- To make this exercise easier: from starting position, pedal the bicycle, but simply hold torso in raised position, without rotation.

Progressions

- Add more reps and sets as you get stronger.

LEGS

EXERCISE 4: SQUAT

You may not have thought about it before, but every time you sit down, you're performing a squat. Maintaining (and improving) muscle strength in the lower body will help you function at your best, with the added benefit of toning your legs and butt. In a survey of 36,000 ACE-certified fitness professionals, the squat was rated number one at shaping and toning the glutes. It's a versatile exercise that can be done with or without weights. Because performing a squat requires the coordinated effort of several muscles, expect to spend some time mastering the techniques of this exercise.

Targets: Thighs (quads and hamstrings), butt (glutes), abs, lower back
Duplicates: Leg Press on a machine

Starting Position

Stand tall in correct posture: feet hips-width apart and firmly planted on the floor, legs straight with knees slightly bent, abs gently contracted, arms at sides, chest slightly lifted, shoulders relaxed and down away from ears, chin parallel to floor, and eyes looking straight ahead. Keep abs pulled up and in toward spine throughout this exercise to protect your lower back, maintain your balance, and help you stay in correct form.

Action

1. As if you were about to sit on a chair, bend slightly forward at the hips, keeping your torso straight, and lower your body by bending your knees, reaching behind you with your butt. At the same time, extend your arms in front of you, parallel to the floor, gently reaching forward with your fingertips. Lower your body until your thighs are parallel with the floor.

2. Pause briefly in this lowered position, then, contracting your glutes and pushing into the floor with your feet, slowly raise

your body back into a standing position.
Do 1 to 3 sets of 8–10 reps.

Technique Tips

- Your weight should be over
  your heels, not over your forefeet.
- Maintaining a straight torso does not
  mean a vertical torso; remember to bend
  slightly forward at the hips as
  you lower your body.
- As you lower yourself into a
  squat, your quads and
  hamstrings are doing
  most of the work. As you
  go lower and your thighs   **Figure 9.4** Squat
  become parallel with the
  floor (and when you push off, returning to starting position), the glutes are more active. Avoid squatting past a parallel position to protect knees from injury.
- Inhale as you lower the body; exhale as you raise it.

Modifications

- If you have balance or strength challenges, don't lower your-self until your thighs are parallel to the floor. You can perform a squat up against the edge of your bed; as you get close to sitting on the bed, raise your body back to starting position. (If you need to just briefly touch the bed with your butt, that's okay, but try to raise yourself before making contact with the bed.) As you get stronger, you can try performing a squat in front of an object lower to the floor, like a chair or couch.
- If you are able to perform a squat but feel just a bit unsteady, practice behind a chair so that you can touch the back of it if needed as you lower and raise your body. Don't grip the back of the chair, just lightly touch it to steady yourself.

Progressions

- Increase the challenge by performing squats more slowly, holding for a few seconds in the lowered position, and raising the body more slowly.

• You can also make squats more difficult by holding dumbbells in each hand (cross arms over chest, resting dumbbells
in front of shoulders) or by wearing a weighted vest.

EXERCISE 5: LUNGE

Strong leg muscles make it possible for us to make lunging
movements when climbing stairs or bending down to pick up
things off the floor. The lunge, rated a very close second as a
top glutes toner and shaper by ACE-certified fitness professionals, is an excellent exercise for lower body strengthening.
Like the squat, this exercise really challenges balance and coordination, so it may take you a few tries to get it right. Begin
with the stationary lunge and progress to the step lunge.

Targets: Thighs (quads and hamstrings), butt (glutes), abs,
back, and calves
Duplicates: Leg Press on a machine

A/Stationary Lunge

Starting Position

Stand tall in correct posture, with your left foot placed on the floor 3–4 feet in front you. Keep your hips square and facing forward, abs contracted, and knees slightly bent. Your weight should be balanced over both feet. Keep abs pulled up and in toward spine throughout this exercise to protect your lower back, maintain your balance, and help you stay in correct form.

Action

1. Simultaneously bend your left knee and lower your right knee toward the floor (your right heel will come off the floor) as you slowly lower your body straight down into a lunge position until your left thigh is parallel with the floor. Your torso will lean forward slightly, but keep your back straight, arms at sides or placed on hips. If you can, pause for 1 or 2 seconds in this position, breathing normally.

Figure 9.5 Lunge

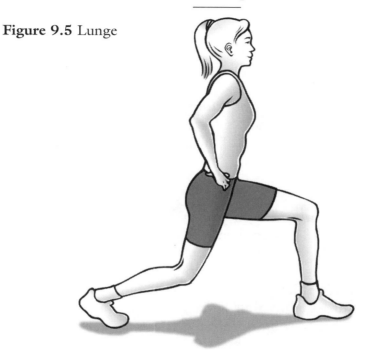

2. Push off against the floor with both feet (you'll feel it in your quads) to return to the starting position. Do 1–3 sets of 8–10 reps. Repeat with opposite starting leg.

B/STEP LUNGE

Starting Position

The starting position is the same as in the standing lunge, except that you'll be standing in correct posture with your feet together, knees slightly bent. Pull abs up and in toward spine.

Action

1. As you step forward with your left foot, planting it on the floor about 2–3 feet in front of you, lower your right knee toward the floor (your right heel will come off the floor) as you lower your body straight down into the lunge position until your left thigh is parallel with the floor. Your torso will lean forward slightly, but keep your back straight, arms at sides or hands resting on hips. If you can, pause for 1 or 2 seconds in this position, breathing normally.

2. Push off against the floor with your left foot to return to the starting position. Do 1–3 sets of 8–10 reps. Repeat with opposite starting leg.

Technique Tips

- Make sure that your knee stays directly over your ankle in your forward leg. Avoid stressing the knee joint; don't let your knee extend past your toes. You may need to take a smaller (or larger) step initially to achieve this.
- Note that your torso will lean forward slightly, but not as much as it does in a squat.
- Don't let the knee of your back leg touch the floor.
- If you're just starting out, don't overdo it. Your butt will be very sore the next day if you do too many lunges on your first day.

Modifications

- If balance is a challenge, practice this exercise next to a chair so that you can touch the back of the chair to steady yourself (try not to hold on to the chair, and don't push against the chair with your hand to return to starting position) if needed.
- If you find it easier, step backward in a lunge. Instead of stepping 2–3 feet forward, step backward, lowering yourself into a lunge position.

- If repeating the lunge on one side of the body several times is too difficult, alternate lunging with each leg.

Progressions

- Work up to taking 3–4 seconds to lower your body, pausing for 1–2 seconds in the lunge position, and taking 3 seconds to raise your body.
- Perform lunge while holding dumbbell in each hand, arms at sides, or while wearing a weighted vest.

BONUS EXERCISE: PULL-UP

The pull-up is really the only effective weight-free exercise to strengthen upper back muscles and biceps. Unfortunately, it's not very accessible: most people can't do pull-ups and don't have pull-up bars in their homes. If you do work out at a health club, or live near a playground equipped with a pull-up bar, and want to try it, here's how:

Targets: Upper back (lats), arms
Duplicates: One-Arm Row with
dumbbell

Starting Position

Jump up or step on a box to reach the bar.

Action

1. Hang on bar, with hands shoulder-width apart or slightly wider, palms facing out.
2. Pull your body up until your chin is level with the bar.
3. Lower your body, but do not fully extend the arms. Do 1–10 reps.

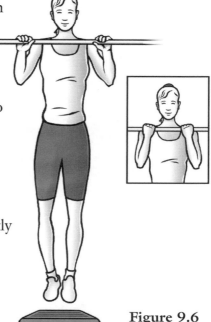

Figure 9.6
Pull-up

Technique Tips

- Keeps abs pulled up and in toward spine, back straight, body vertical.
- Don't lock elbows or arch back.
- Do this exercise after push-up.
- This version works the back and triceps; to emphasize the biceps and back, change hand grip so that palms face you. *(See inset to Figure 9.6.)*

Modification

- If you can't pull yourself up, start in the raised position of step 2, and hold for 10–20 seconds.

10 | Small Weights, Big Gains: The Dumbbell Workout

BUILDING BALANCED STRENGTH

Incorporating dumbbells into your strength training exercises is an effective and efficient way to add variety to your fitness repertoire, make new strength gains, and strengthen both sides of the body equally, addressing strength imbalances and deficiencies and improving balance and coordination.

DUMBBELL EXERCISES

This workout consists of both exercises using weights and using body weight as resistance. Like the previous workout, this routine contains primarily compound, multi-joint exercises, plus a few isolation exercises such as the biceps curl, overhead triceps extension, and triceps kickback to strengthen and tone smaller muscles. You'll notice that holding weights makes balancing and maintaining coordination more difficult. Remember to stabilize the torso before lifting by pulling your abdominal muscles up and in toward your spine.

SELECTING YOUR DUMBBELLS

Select a weight that's appropriate for your strength and skill level. It's a good idea to begin with a weight that's slightly too easy to lift so that you can focus on performing the exercises in correct form. After a few workouts, switch to a weight that you can lift at least 8 times, but begins to cause muscle fatigue and loss of form if you lift it more than 10 times. Most people can begin with 3- or 5-pound dumbbells.

You won't be using the same weight in every exercise because some parts of the body are stronger than others. For example, when making a compound movement like the chest press that involves two joints and several large muscles, you'll be able to lift more weight than you would performing a single-joint isolation exercise like the biceps curl. You'll probably be able to use the most weight in lower body exercises since the quads are the strongest muscles in the body. Pay attention to these differences, and adjust your weights accordingly.

FORM AND TECHNIQUE

It's worth repeating: Prepare yourself for exercise by reviewing the guidelines, techniques, and health cautions described throughout this book, including the six techniques for performing strength training exercises correctly, listed in Chapter 7.

ORDER OF EXERCISES

After a five- to ten-minute warmup that includes light aerobic activity and stretching all of the major muscle groups, perform the exercises in the order they appear:

1. Dumbbell Press or Dumbbell Fly
2. Superperson
3. One-Arm Row
4. Shoulder Press
5. Biceps Curl
6. Overhead Triceps Extension or Triceps Kickback
7. Vertical Crunch
8. One-Legged Squat
9. Directional Lunge

After four to eight weeks, you can switch the order of the exercises, performing lower body exercises before upper body exercises, with the abs exercise in the middle or at the end of the workout. Perform biceps curl before either triceps exercise, and both arm exercises after the other upper body exercises. Follow this workout by stretching all of the major muscle groups again.

CHEST

For variety's sake, there are two chest exercises listed here. It's not necessary to do both; select one each time you do this workout.

EXERCISE 1A: DUMBBELL PRESS

Strengthening chest muscles helps you develop the upper body strength you need to make pushing movements, like pressing open heavy doors.

Targets: Chest (pectorals), shoulders
Duplicates: Bench Press with free weights, Chest Press on machine

Starting Position

Lie on the floor with knees bent, feet a few inches apart (but no wider than hips-width), and heels about a foot away from buttocks. You should have a small natural curve in your lower back, creating a small space between your back and the floor. Holding a dumbell in each hand, extend your arms in line with your shoulders. With your upper arms resting against the floor, bend your arms so that your hands line up vertically over your elbows. Keep abs pulled up and in toward spine throughout this exercise to protect your lower back and maintain neutral spine. Inhale before initiating movement.

Action

1. As you exhale, extend your arms, pressing the dumbbells straight up toward the ceiling. Pause for 1 or 2 seconds. As you inhale, lower your arms to the starting position. Do 1 to 3 sets of 8–10 reps.

Technique Tips

- Raise and lower weights using slow, controlled movements. Resist the urge to rely on momentum or to arch your back when you become tired.

Figure 10.1a Dumbbell Press

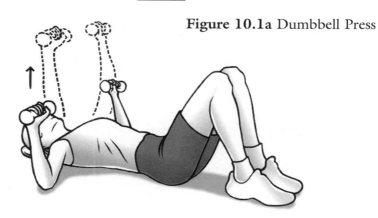

- Do not lock your elbows when you extend your arms. Raised dumbbells should line up over shoulders.
- Do not hold the weights tightly; maintain a loose but stable grip.

Modification

- Start with 1-pound weights if necessary to develop coordination and strength.

Progressions

- Gradually increase the weight of dumbbells in 2- to 3-pound increments as you are able.

EXERCISE 1B: DUMBBELL FLY

Flys (sometimes spelled flyes) also strengthen chest muscles but challenge them with a different motion. Because this movement isolates the chest muscles, you will need to use lighter dumbbells than you used for the dumbbell press.

Targets: Chest (pectorals)
Duplicates: Cable machine

Starting Position

Lie on the floor with knees bent, feet a few inches apart (but no wider than hips-width), and heels about a foot away from buttocks. You should have a small natural curve in your lower back, creating a small space between your back and the floor.

Figure 10.1b Dumbbell Fly

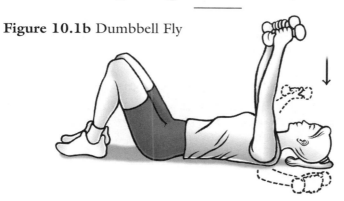

Holding a dumbbell in each hand, extend arms vertically, placing palms together and holding arms in a slightly bent but fixed position. Keep abs pulled up and in toward spine throughout this exercise to protect your lower back and maintain neutral spine.

Action

1. As you inhale, slowly lower your arms toward the floor, leading the movement with your weights, as if you're a bird opening up your wings. Continue lowering weights until you feel a stretch across your chest and the front of your shoul-

ders. Stop just before your arms touch the floor. Pause in this position for 1 to 2 seconds.

2. As you exhale, slowly raise your hands, sweeping your arms back into the starting position as if you're embracing someone. Do 1 to 3 sets of 8–10 reps. *(See Figure 10.1b.)*

Technique Tips

- Keep arms straight, but don't lock your elbows.
- Do not touch weights to floor.
- Raise and lower weights using slow, controlled movements. Resist the urge to rely on momentum or to arch your back when you become tired.
- Do not hold the weights tightly; maintain a loose but stable grip.

Modification

- Start with 1-pound weights if necessary to develop coordination and strength.

Progressions

- Gradually increase the weight of dumbbells in 2- to 3-pound increments as you are able.

BACK

EXERCISE 2: SUPERPERSON

The superperson adds more intensity to the back extension from the previous workout by having you extend your arms in front of your body while simultaneously performing a leg lift. This weight-free move is one of the most effective ways to address lower back strength and can be safer than some free-weight alternatives.

    Targets: Lower back (erector spinae)
Duplicates: Back Extension on machine, Stiff-Legged Dead Lift with barbell

Starting Position

Lie facedown with arms extended in front of body and in line with shoulders, hands palms down, legs together. Keep your abs pulled up and in toward the spine, and your hips and pubic bone pressed to the floor. Take an inhaling breath before initiating movement.

Action

1. With an exhaling breath, raise both your chest and feet 3–5 inches off of the floor as if you're flying through the air like Superman.

   As you raise your chest, keep arms extended, parallel, and in line with your ears. Resist the urge to scrunch your shoulders; keep them pulled down away from your ears. Visualize your spine extending from your tailbone out the top of your head. Keep your neck long, straight, and relaxed. Pause in this position for 1 to 2 seconds, breathing normally.

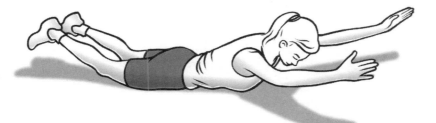

Figure 10.2a Superperson

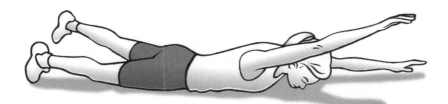

Figure 10.2b Swimming

2. Slowly lower chest and legs to floor. Do 1 to 3 sets of 8–10 reps. (Note: Follow this exercise with an effective lower back stretch.)

Technique Tips

- Don't pull your head back with extension; maintaining eye contact with the floor will help you keep your neck straight and your head in the correct position.
- Maintain abs to spine and contract your glutes (by squeezing together your buttocks) to help protect the lower back.
- Avoid extending your back too far to reduce injury risk. The height you are able to raise your chest and feet from the floor will vary from person to person—use 3 to 5 inches as a guideline.
- Lead the movement with your chest, not with your arms. Resist the urge to use your arms for momentum when you get tired.
- You can put a folded towel under the front of your hips to help reduce pressure on lower back.

Modification

- If this version is too difficult, begin in starting position and go swimming; instead of raising chest, simultaneously raise your right arm and left leg 4–5 inches from the floor, keeping chin touching the floor. Hold position for a few seconds, inhaling and exhaling slowly and deliberately. Repeat with left arm and right leg. Do 1–3 sets of 8–10 reps. *(See Figure 10.2b.)*

MID-BACK

EXERCISE 3: ONE-ARM ROW

If your posture isn't exactly what it could be, this exercise will help you stop slouching and get a better-looking back. Having a strong back is important for overall core strength.

Targets: Mid-back (lats and rhomboids)
Duplicates: Lat Pull-down on a machine

Starting Position

Holding a dumbbell in your right hand, stand in a semi-lunge position, with your left leg forward, thigh approaching parallel to the floor, knee aligned over ankle, and your right leg extended behind you. Rotate your right foot slightly to the right for a more comfortable stance. Bend forward at the hips and rest your left forearm across your thigh just above your knee, but don't lean into your arm for support. Allow your right arm to hang at your side. Keep abs pulled up and in toward spine throughout this exercise to protect your lower back and maintain neutral spine. Your right ankle, right knee, hips, shoulders, and ears should form a straight line. Inhale before initiating movement.

Action

1. As you exhale, slowly pull the dumbbell straight up, keeping your elbow close to your body, until your upper arm passes the line of your torso. Use your back muscle to initiate the movement before your arm muscles become engaged. Pause

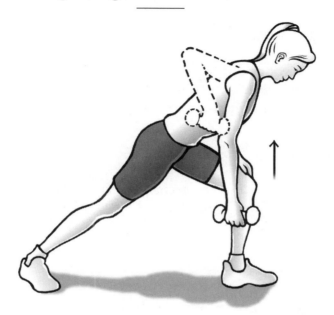

Figure 10.3 One-Arm Row

for a second or two when you reach the end of your range of motion, then slowly lower dumbbell toward floor. Do 1–3 sets of 8–10 reps on each side of body.

Technique Tips

- Don't let your head (or shoulder of working arm) droop forward; don't lean into your resting arm for support.
- Exhale as you raise the dumbbell; inhale as you lower it.

Modification

- Perform row sitting in a chair, with a pillow on your lap, knees aligned over ankles. Bend forward at the hips approximately 45°, keeping torso straight.

Progression

- Holding a dumbbell in each hand and standing with feet shoulders-width apart, knees slightly bent, bend forward at the hips (to about a 45° angle). Slowly raise dumbbells, keeping arms close to body, until your upper arms pass the line of your torso. Pause for 1 to 2 seconds; slowly lower to starting position.

SHOULDERS

EXERCISE 4: SHOULDER PRESS

Strengthening your shoulders helps shape and define your arms. Women battling bra bulge also use this exercise to firm up the area under the armpits. Strong shoulders come in handy when you have to put away a heavy box on the top shelf of your closet.

Targets: Shoulders (anterior and medial deltoids), triceps
Duplicates: Shoulder Press with barbell or Military Press on a machine

Starting Position

Stand in correct posture with feet hips-width apart, holding a dumbbell in each hand just above each shoulder. Keep abs pulled up and in toward spine throughout this exercise to protect your lower back and maintain neutral spine.

Action

1. Slowly extend arms, pushing dumbbells straight toward the ceiling. Pause for 1 or 2 seconds, then slowly lower dumbbells, returning to starting position. Do 1–3 sets of 8–10 reps.

Technique Tips

- Do not lock your elbows when you extend arms.
- Inhale as you lower weights; exhale as you raise them.
- Maintain correct posture; don't allow your shoulders to scrunch up with movement or your back to arch.

Modification

- Perform press sitting in a chair in correct posture, with knees aligned over ankles.

Progressions

- Gradually increase the amount of weight used.

Figure 10.4
Shoulder Press

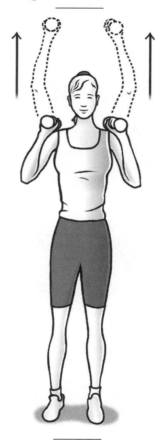

ARMS

EXERCISE 5: BICEPS CURL

Biceps are everybody's favorite "show me your muscles" muscle. Strengthening biceps can help you achieve definition in your arms and give you more power when making pulling movements.

Targets: Arms (biceps)
Duplicates: Biceps Curl on a machine or with a barbell

Starting Position

Holding a dumbbell in your right hand, stand with feet hips-width apart, arms at sides, right palm facing forward. Keep abs pulled up and in toward spine throughout this exercise to protect your lower back and maintain neutral spine.

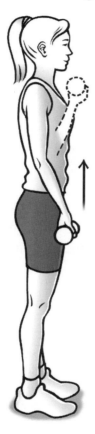

Action

1. Pressing your right elbow to your side, slowly raise the dumbbell toward your right shoulder, squeezing biceps at the top of the lift. Pause for 1 to 2 seconds when you reach the end of your range of motion (you should not touch weights to shoulders), then slowly lower the weight to the starting position. Do 1–3 sets of 8–10 reps. Repeat with left arm.

Technique Tips

- Maintain correct posture. Don't allow your shoulders to scrunch up. Keep wrists straight.

Figure 10.5 Biceps Curl

- Work your muscles as you raise *and* lower the dumbbells; don't rely on momentum to lift or lower weights.
- Inhale as you lower weight; exhale as you raise it.

Modification

- Perform curls sitting on the edge of a chair in correction posture, knees aligned above ankles.

Progressions

- For variety, curl both arms at the same time, or alternate between each arm.
- Gradually increase weight, or perform single biceps curl while balancing on one leg (don't lock knee of supporting leg, and switch legs when you work the opposite arm).

EXERCISE 6A: OVERHEAD TRICEPS EXTENSION

The triceps muscles extend the arm and are used in all pushing motions. These triceps exercises will help you firm up the flab on the underside of your arms. Two versions are included here for variety's sake. You can choose one each time you work out.

Targets: Arm (triceps)
Duplicates: Triceps Extension on a machine

Starting Position

Holding a dumbbell in your right hand, stand with feet hips-width apart, with your right arm extended vertically and bent so that the dumbbell is behind your head. Keep abs pulled up and in toward spine throughout this exercise to protect your lower back and maintain neutral spine.

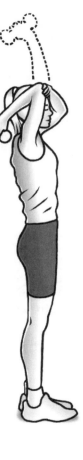

Action

1. Keeping your right elbow close to your head, slowly push the dumbbell toward the ceiling, extending your right arm. You may find it helpful to gently hold and support your extended arm with your left hand. Pause for 1 to 2 seconds before slowly lowering the dumbbell to starting position. Do 1–3 sets of 8–10 reps. Repeat with left arm.

Technique Tips

- Don't allow your shoulders to scrunch up; keep them relaxed and down away from ears.

Figure 10.6a Overhead Triceps Extension

- Don't lock your elbow when you extend your lifting arm.
- Keep elbow of lifting arm pointing up and close to your head; don't allow your arm to fall forward. Keep wrists straight.

Modification

- This can be done sitting on the edge of a chair (as in seated biceps curl).

Progressions

- Gradually increase weights.
- Work the triceps while using a different stance *(see next exercise)*.

EXERCISE 6B: TRICEPS KICKBACK

Starting Position

Stand in a semi-lunge position, with your left leg forward, thigh approaching parallel to the floor, knee aligned over ankle, and your right leg extended behind you. Rotate your right foot slightly to the right for a more comfortable stance. Bend forward at the hips and rest your left forearm across your thigh just above your knee, but don't lean into your arm for support. Keeping your upper right arm pressed against your body, parallel to the floor, allow your right hand to hang below the elbow, holding a dumbbell. Keep abs pulled up and in toward spine throughout this exercise to protect your lower back and maintain neutral spine. Your right ankle, right knee, hips, shoulders, and ears should form a straight line. Inhale before initiating movement.

Action

1. With an exhaling breath, slowly push the dumbbell behind you, extending your arm and keeping your elbow pressed

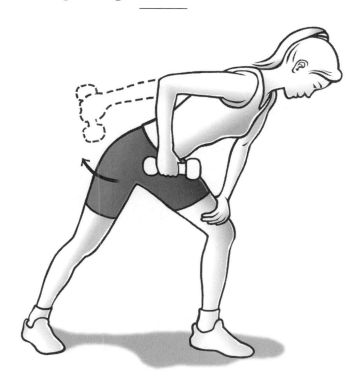

Figure 10.6b Triceps Kickback

against your body. Pause for 1 to 2 seconds in this position, then slowly return to starting position. Do 1–3 sets of 8–10 reps. Repeat with left arm. *(See Figure 10.6b.)*

Technique Tips

- Don't rely on momentum; control the movement through both the lifting and lowering phase of the exercise.
- Inhale as you return to staring position; exhale as you initiate movement.
- Maintain alignment; don't allow your head (or shoulder of working arm) to droop forward.

Modification

- See modifications for standing triceps exercise on page 137.

Progressions

- Gradually increase weights.

ABS

EXERCISE 7: VERTICAL CRUNCH

This variation on the crunch is another abs exercise given a top-rating by the ACE.

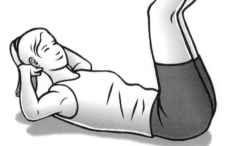

Targets: Abs (rectus abdominis, internal and external obliques, and transverse abdominis)

Duplicates: Crunch or Abs Curl on machine

Starting Position

Lie on your back with your knees bent, feet flat on the floor, fingertips placed against the sides of your head, just behind the ears. Pull your abs up and in toward your spine,

Figure 10.7 Vertical Crunch

and maintain contraction throughout exercise. Slowly raise your feet in the air, one at a time, until your legs are perpendicular to your torso. Inhale before initiating any movement.

Action

1. As you exhale, slowly raise your upper body until your shoulder blades are no longer touching the floor. You'll feel the "crunch" of your abs contracting as your rib cage moves closer to your pelvis. Lower your body to the floor slowly, controlling the movement with your abs. Keep looking up as you perform each crunch to prevent bending your neck forward. Repeat 8–10 times, adding more reps (and sets) as you can.

Technique Tips

- Cross your legs at the ankles to help improve stability if necessary.
- Initiate movement from the abs, and lift the chest, shoulders, neck, and head as one unit. Do not pull on your head or bend your neck forward.

- Try to keep your legs still.
- Try to maintain neutral spine.

Modification

- If this move is too challenging, try doing the crunch with knees bent, lower legs parallel to the floor (and if necessary, you can rest your lower legs on the seat of a chair).

Progressions

- If you can, include rotation in your crunch, alternating lifting and rotating to each side. Add more reps to each set as you get stronger.

LEGS

EXERCISE 8: ONE-LEGGED SQUAT

One-legged squats turn up the heat on lower body muscles by challenging balance. You'll feel the burn in your quads while you're holding the squat and in your glutes following the workout.

Targets: Thighs (quads and hamstrings), butt (glutes), and abs

Duplicates: Leg Press on machine and Squat with a barbell

Starting Position

Stand in correct posture, with feet hips-width apart, arms extended straight in front of you, parallel to the floor. Pull abs up and in toward spine to protect lower back, maintain neutral spine, and aid in balance. Lift right foot off floor a few inches, extending right leg in front of you.

Action

1. Balancing on your left leg, slowly lower yourself into a squat position. You won't be able to lean as far forward as you did in a two-legged squat or lower yourself as far. Pause for 1 to 2 seconds, then contract your glutes (i.e., squeeze your buttocks together), press into the floor with your left foot, and slowly raise yourself into starting position. Do 1–3 sets of 8–10 reps. Repeat with right leg.

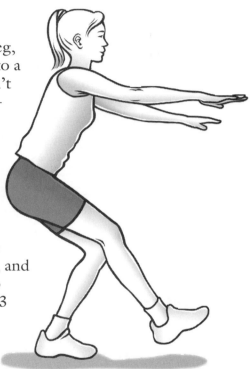

Figure 10.8 One-Legged Squat

Technique Tips

- Unlike in a regular squat, your knees will be over your toes, not your ankles, when you squat. And your thigh will not be parallel to the floor; most people can't lower themselves that far.
- Don't lock the knee of the extended leg.
- Complete all sets with right leg before working left leg.
- Inhale as you squat; exhale as you return to starting position.

Modification

- Perform next to a chair, desk, or countertop if you feel unsteady.

Progressions

- Do more reps, more sets, slow down the pace, hold small weights (at sides or in front of shoulders), or wear a weighted vest.

EXERCISE 9: DIRECTIONAL LUNGE

Like the lunges in the previous workout, this lunge is a challenging exercise designed to build lower body strength and improve balance and coordination. This, too, will take a bit of practice to master.

Targets: Thighs (quads and hamstrings), butt (glutes), abs
Duplicates: Leg Press on machine

Starting Position

Stand in correct posture, with your feet hips-width apart, arms hanging at your sides or hands resting on hips. Keep abs pulled up and in toward spine throughout this exercise to protect lower back and aid in balance. Visualize that you are standing in the center of a clock, and your goal is to perform a lunge with your right foot touching the numbers 1, 2, and 3, and then your left foot stepping on 11, 10, and 9.

Action

1. Keeping your feet parallel to each other, hips square and facing forward, step forward into a lunge position, placing your right foot at 1 o'clock. The thigh of your right leg should be parallel to the floor, knee over ankle, body straight and bent slightly forward at hips. Your left leg will be bent, toward the floor, with the heel of your left foot coming off the floor. Pause in this position for 1 to 2 seconds.

2. Return to starting position by pressing off the floor with right foot. You'll also contract your abs and glutes to help you return to the starting position.

3. Repeat the lunge at 2, then 3 o'clock positions. Then repeat with left leg, lunging toward the 11, 10, and 9 o'clock positions. Do 1–3 sets of 8–10 reps for each number.

Technique Tips

- Notice that because of the angles of movement, your legs won't align exactly the same way as in a basic lunge. As you

Figure 10.9 Directional Lunge

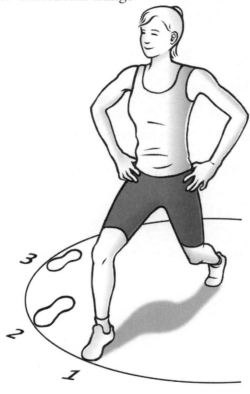

lunge in either direction away from 12 o'clock, your knee may not line up exactly over your ankle, but in some cases, over your toes.

- Try to keep your feet parallel, hips square.

Modification

- If it's too difficult to move from position to position, practice lunging to 1 o'clock with right foot and 9 o'clock with left foot, gradually adding the second and third positions.

Progressions

- Add reps, go slower, hold hand weights, or wear a weighted vest.

11 | Combo Moves: A Mini Power Workout

INCREASING INTENSITY

Once you've mastered the previous two workouts and you're ready for new challenges, you can combine upper and lower body exercises to create powerful combo moves that crank up the intensity of your workouts.

BENEFITS OF COMBO MOVES

Combo moves are true all-body exercises that work several muscle groups at once; they're ideal for building the type of functional strength you need to perform everyday tasks. Exercising the upper and lower body at the same time makes your muscles and your cardiovascular system work harder, so you'll burn more calories and improve your fitness level. In addition, these time-saving moves train the body to integrate limb and torso movement to build balanced strength.

FORM AND TECHNIQUE

These dynamic moves are much more challenging than the exercises in the previous workouts. Maintaining your balance and performing the moves in correct form will be very difficult, so you shouldn't attempt these exercises until you're strong enough and coordinated enough to perform them correctly. Pay attention to correct technique to avoid straining your lower back.

Here are a few technique tips to keep in mind:

- Start with lighter weights that you used in the previous workout; increase resistance gradually.

- Keep your abs pulled up and in toward your spine throughout each exercise to protect your lower back and aid in balance.
- Perform the exercises in one fluid movement. Initially, you may have to break the moves down into two moves as you learn how to do them.

How to Use the Exercises

The four moves in this chapter can be used as a mini-workout on days you're pressed for time, or individual moves can be incorporated into weight-free or dumbbell workouts to replace corresponding upper and lower body exercises. When adding these moves to another workout, perform them first.

Order of Exercises

After a five- to ten-minute warm-up that includes light aerobic activity and stretching all the major muscle groups, perform the exercises in the order they appear:

1. Squat Press
2. Lunge and Biceps Curl
3. Side Lunge Reach
4. Walking Push-up

Follow these moves with an adequate stretching session, making sure to address lower back muscles.

EXERCISE 1: SQUAT PRESS

Targets: Thighs (quads and hamstrings), butt (glutes), shoulders, abs

Starting Position

Holding a dumbbell in each hand, just above each shoulder, palms facing each other, stand tall in correct posture with feet hips-width apart. Pull abs up and in toward spine to protect lower back, maintain neutral spine, and aid in balance.

Action

1. Simultaneously lower your body into a squat, until thighs are parallel with the floor, and raise the dumbbells straight into the air. Pause briefly, then simultaneously lower weights and stand up, returning to starting position. Do 1–3 sets of 8–10 reps.

Technique Tips

- Remember to lean forward slightly, bending at the hips and keeping your back straight as you squat. Because of the dumbbells you won't lean forward as far as you would in a regular squat.
- Knees should be aligned over toes.
- Don't forget to breathe. Inhale as you lower the body; exhale as you raise it.

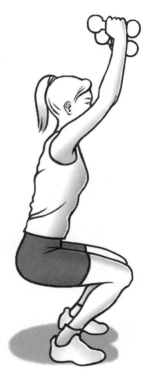

Figure 11.1 Squat Press

Modification

- If this move is too difficult, break it down into two moves. First, holding weights in front of shoulders, perform a squat. When you return to starting position, perform a shoulder press.

EXERCISE 2: LUNGE AND BICEPS CURL

Targets: Thighs (quads and hamstrings), butt (glutes), biceps, abs

Starting Position

Holding a dumbbell in each hand, arms at sides, palms facing thighs, stand tall in correct posture, feet hips-width apart. Pull abs up and in toward spine to protect lower back, maintain neutral spine, and aid in balance. *(See Figure 11.2a.)*

Combo Moves: A Mini Power Workout

Figure 11.2a

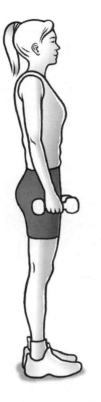

Figure 11.2b Lunge and Biceps Curl

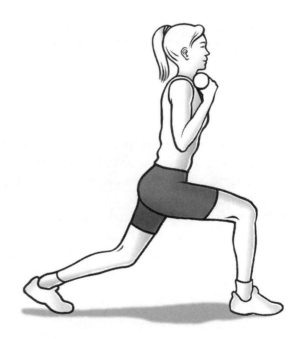

Action

1. Pressing elbows to sides, perform a biceps curl with each arm as you step forward with your right leg into a lunge position. *(See Figure 11.2b.)*
2. Lower the weights back down to your sides as you press off with your right foot, returning to a standing position. Do 1–3 sets of 8–10 reps. Repeat with opposite leg.

Technique Tips

- As you raise dumbbells to perform the curl, first rotate dumbbells outward so that your palms face your shoulders as you raise the weights. Keep elbows pressed to sides, wrists straight.
- When you step forward with your right leg, also bend your left leg, lowering left knee toward the floor (your left heel will come off the floor). In the lunge position, your right thigh should be parallel with the floor, knee over ankle.

Modification

- If this move is too difficult, break it down into two moves. First perform a biceps curl, then the lunge (while holding weights in front of shoulders or with arms at sides).

EXERCISE 3: SIDE LUNGE REACH

Targets: Chest, upper back, hips, thighs (abductors, adductors, quads, hamstrings), butt (glutes), shoulders

Starting Position

Stand tall in correct posture, balanced on your right leg, with your right arm extended straight above your right shoulder, holding a dumbbell. Pull abs up and in toward spine to protect lower back, maintain neutral spine, and aid in balance. *(See Figure 11.3a.)*

Action

1. As you perform a side lunge, stepping out with your left foot, reach down to your left ankle with the dumbbell. *(See Figure 11.3b.)* Then simultaneously press into your left foot and raise the weight back across the front of the body and into the raised position above your right shoulder, returning to the starting position. Do 1–3 sets of 8–10 reps. Repeat on opposite side of the body.

Technique Tips

- Don't rely on momentum.
- Your butt will be sore after this one!

Combo Moves: A Mini Power Workout

Figure 11.3a

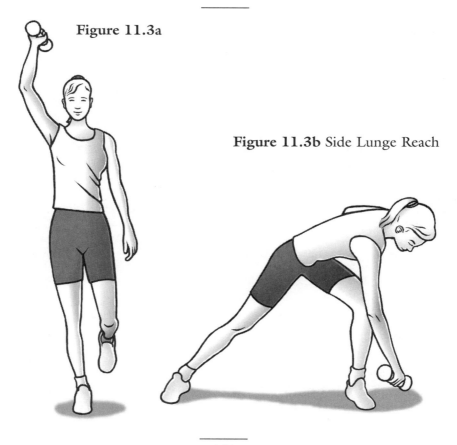

Figure 11.3b Side Lunge Reach

EXERCISE 4: WALKING PUSH-UP

Targets: Abs, back, hips, chest, and shoulders

Starting Position

From kneeling on hands and knees, get into a raised push-up position, with legs together, but put hands right next to each other instead of underneath shoulders. Pull abs up and in toward spine to protect lower back, maintain neutral spine, and aid in balance.

Action

1. With left hand and left foot, step out to the left about a foot, then do a push-up. When you return to the raised position, step hand and foot back to starting position.
2. Next, with right hand and right foot, step out to the right about a foot, then do a push-up. Return to starting position once body is raised. Do as many reps as you can on both sides of body.

Figure 11.4 Walking Push-up

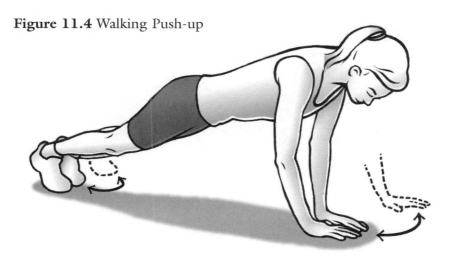

Technique Tips

- Keep back straight, spine in neutral, head in line with spine.
- Don't forget to breathe. Inhale as you lower your body; exhale as you push up.

12 | Conclusion: A Lifetime of Fitness

IMPROVING STRENGTH AND HEALTH

Now that you've learned the basics, you're ready to get started in a strength training program that will help you improve your strength, balance, coordination, flexibility, and posture. Hopefully, you've gained a greater understanding of why strength training is an important exercise and more confidence about taking on a new challenge.

Conclusion: A lifetime of Fitness

REAPING THE BENEFITS

Once you've had a few weeks to practice the exercises in this book, you'll start to see how strength training can make you stronger, leaner, and fitter. After a few more weeks, and some hard work, you'll even be able to see changes in your appearance.

KEEP LEARNING

Reading more about strength training, taking some strength training classes, and working with an experienced and certified personal trainer every three to six months to reassess and adjust your workouts are all great ways to help you stay on track and continue making progress.

GET STRONG; STAY HEALTHY

With strength training as part of your overall health and fitness plan, along with regular aerobic exercise, flexibility training, and a healthy diet, you'll not only get stronger, but you'll have more energy, greater stamina, and a healthier body.

Glossary

Barbell

A weighted bar approximately four feet in length, on which weighted iron plates are attached near both ends. Used in weight-lifting exercises. *See* illustration on page 17.

Body mechanics

Refers to ergonomic movements. When practicing strength training exercises, it's important to maintain correct posture and body alignment.

167

GLOSSARY

Compound movements Also called compound exercises. *See* multi-joint.

Concentric phase The initial or "lifting" phase of a strength training exercise.

Dumbbells Handheld weights, smaller duplicates of barbells. *See* illustration on page 17.

Eccentric phase The second phase in a strength training exercise in which the weight is returned to the starting position.

Ergonomic The correct alignment of the body during movement.

Extension Extending or straightening a joint.

Flexion Bending a joint.

Isolation movements

Also called isolation exercises. *See* single-joint.

Large muscles

Large muscles are primarily responsible for supporting and moving the body. Example: hip, leg, chest, and shoulder muscles.

Moderate intensity

Working at 55 to 65 percent of your maximum heart rate. In other words, you want to break a sweat but still be able to carry on a conversation with an exercise partner.

Multi-joint

A multi-joint exercise or movement involves more than one joint. For example: the push-up, which involves elbow and shoulder joints.

Single-joint

A single-joint exercise or movement involves only one joint. For example: the biceps curl, which involves the elbow joint.

Small muscles

Small muscles are smaller in size than large muscles and support larger muscles in stabilization and movement. Examples: biceps and calves.

Resources

STRENGTH TRAINING EQUIPMENT

While researching this book, I used a variety of strength training equipment, provided by the following companies.

Reebok International, Ltd.
1895 JW Foster Boulevard
Canton, MA 02021
800-Reebok1 (733-2651)
www.reebok.com
Sample product: weighted vest

RESOURCES

The Nautilus Group
1886 Prairie Way
Louisville, CO 80027
800-864-1270
www.nautilusgroup.com
www.schwinnfitness.com
www.stairmaster.com
Sample products: dumbbells, barbells, weight machines

NIKE, Inc.
One Bowerman Drive
P.O. Box 4027
Beaverton, OR 97005
800-806-6453
www.niketown.com
Sample products: dumbbells, workout gloves, wrist and ankle
weights, resistance bands

Resources

Probell
1693 W. Hamlin Road
Rochester, MI 48309-3312
877-777-6235
www.probell.com
Sample product: adjustable weight chrome dumbbells

AquaBells Travel Weights
3231 W. Boone Avenue, Unit 3
Spokane, WA 99201
800-987-6892
www.aquabells.com
Sample products: water-filled dumbbells and ankle weights for
    travel

TMG Fit
The McCorry Group, Inc.
105 Price Avenue
Berwyn, PA 19312
800-698-1498
www.tmgfit.com
Sample products: weighted vest, wrist and ankle weights

RESOURCES

Ivanko Barbell Company
P.O. Box 1470
San Pedro, CA 90733
310-514-1155
www.ivanko.com
Sample products: dumbbells, barbells, commercial weight
   machines

EDUCATION/INFORMATION

For more information on fitness programs, types of exercises,
and health tips, contact the following organizations.

The American College of Sports Medicine
317-637-9200
www.acsm.org

The American Council on Exercise
800-825-3636
www.acefitness.org

Resources

The American Senior Fitness Association
800-243-1478
www.seniorfitness.net

The National Strength and Conditioning Association
800-815-6826
www.nsca-lift.org

IDEAFit
6190 Cornerstone Court East, Suite 204
San Diego, CA 92121-3773
858-535-8979
www.ideafit.com

For information on which activities burn the most calories, check out www.caloriecounter.org.

For more information about Erika Dillman's Little Fitness Books series, vist her Web site at www.littlefitnessbooks.com.

Notes

CHAPTER THREE

1. Schwinn Fitness Facts. www.schwinnfitness.com.

2. Shaffer, Alyssa L. "Strength in Numbers: Need a Reason to Start Lifting Dumbbells or Your Bodyweight?" *Sports Illustrated for Women*, March 1, 2001, vol. 3, issue 2, pages 84+.

3. Schwinn Fitness Facts. www.schwinnfitness.com.

4. Nelson, Miriam, Ph.D. *Strong Women Stay Slim* (New York: Bantam Books, 1998). Pages 3–28.

5. Bean, Adam. "Burn Fat Faster." *Runner's World*, November 2001, vol. 36, issue 11, page 50.

6. Williams, Vanessa Selene. "Resistance Is Not Futile." *American Fitness*, September 2001, vol. 19, issue 5, page 27.

7. "Lower Blood Pressure by Exercising and Losing Weight." *Strength and Conditioning*, June 2002.

8. Shaffer, Alyssa L. "Strength in Numbers: Need a Reason to Start Lifting Dumbbells or Your Bodyweight?" *Sports Illustrated for Women*, March 1, 2001, vol. 3, issue 2, pages 84+.

9. Schwinn Fitness Facts. www.schwinnfitness.com.

10. Shaffer, Alyssa L. "Strength in Numbers: Need a Reason to Start Lifting Dumbbells or Your Bodyweight?" *Sports Illustrated for Women*, March 1, 2001, vol. 3, issue 2, pages 84+.

11. Shaffer, Alyssa L. "Strength in Numbers: Need a Reason to Start Lifting Dumbbells or Your Bodyweight?" *Sports Illustrated for Women*, March 1, 2001, vol. 3, issue 2, pages 84+.

12 Williams, Vanessa Selene. "Resistance Is Not Futile." *American Fitness*, September 2001, vol. 19, issue 5, page 27.

13. Williams, Vanessa Selene. "Resistance Is Not Futile." *American Fitness*, September 2001, vol. 19, issue 5, page 27.

14. Gorman, Christine, and Miriam Nelson, Ph.D. "Muscle Power: Why You Should Get Stronger." *Time*, July 22, 2002, vol. 160, issue 4, G9.

15. Droste, Therese. "Adding a Little Iron to Your Life: Strength Training Programs Aim to Help Seniors Stay Independent by Maintaining Mobility." *The Washington Post*, January 23, 2001, T11.

Notes

Chapter Four

1. American Council on Exercise fact sheet. www.acefitness.org.

Chapter Five

1. Chart compiled from information in:
    Calais-Germain, Blandine. *Anatomy of Movement* (Seattle, Wash.: Eastland Press, 1993). Sprague, Ken. *The Gold's Gym Book of Strength Training.* (New York: Perigree, 1994). Thibodeau, Gary A., and Catherine Parker Anthony. *Structure & Function of the Body* (St. Louis, Mo.: Times Mirror/Mosby College Publishing, 1988).

Chapter Six

1. Westcott, Wayne, Ph.D. "Research on Advanced Strength Training." Naturalstrength.com, April 15, 2000.
2. Westcott, Wayne, Ph.D. "Research on Advanced Strength Training." Naturalstrength.com, April 15, 2000.
3. Adapted from information on www.iDEAFIT.com.
4. The National Strength and Conditioning Association. *The NSCA*

Quick Series Guide to Basic Weight Training (Colorado Springs, Colo.: NSCA, 1997).

CHAPTER SEVEN

1. Adapted from information in *Sculpting Her Body Perfect* by Brad Schoenfeld (Champaign, Ill.: Human Kinetics, 2000).

CHAPTER EIGHT

1. Westcott, Wayne, Ph.D., and Jane Guy. "A Physical Revolution." *IDEA Today*, 1996, vol. 14, no. 9, pages 56–58.

2. Pollock, Michael L., Ph.D., et al. "The Recommended Quantity and Quality of Exercise for Developing and Maintaining Cardiorespiratory and Muscular Fitness, and Flexibility in Healthy Adults." *Medicine & Science in Sports & Exercise*, June 1998, vol. 30, no. 6.

Bibliography

Andes, Karen. *A Woman's Book of Strength* (New York: Perigree, 1995).

Brooks, Douglas. *Effective Strength Training* (Champaign, Ill.: Human Kinetics, 2001).

Coleman, Lori. *Beginning Strength Training* (Minneapolis, Minn.: Lerner, 1998).

Jarrell, Steve. *Working Out With Weights* (New York: Arco, 1978).

Nelson, Miriam, Ph.D. *Strong Women Stay Slim* (New York: Bantam, 1998).

Nelson, Miriam, Ph.D. *Strong Women, Strong Bones* (New York: G.P. Putnam's Sons, 2000).

BIBLIOGRAPHY

Nelson, Miriam, Ph.D. *Strong Women and Men Beat Arthritis* (New York: G.P. Putnam's Sons, 2002).

Pearl, Bill. *Getting Stronger* (Bolinas, Calif.: Shelter Publications, 2001).

Pollock, Michael L., Ph.D., et al. "The Recommended Quantity and Quality of Exercise for Developing and Maintaining Cardiorespiratory and Muscular Fitness, and Flexibility in Healthy Adults." *Medicine & Science in Sports & Exercise*, vol. 30, no. 6, June 1998.

Sprague, Ken. *The Gold's Gym Book of Strength Training* (New York: Perigree, 1994).

Index

INDEX

Index

INDEX

Index

Index

Index

INDEX

more . . .

THE LITTLE ABS WORKOUT BOOK

Everyone wants killer abs. Now you can learn how to trim your torso and tighten your stomach for that six-pack look and greater overall strength! This book's progressive training plan will help you gradually restore function, strength, and endurance to abs and back muscles; improve your posture and balance; reduce the risk of lower back pain; and achieve the flat, chiseled abdomen that looks so great. Complete with easy-to-follow instructions and detailed illustrations, it's the perfect training companion.

THE LITTLE FOOT CARE BOOK

If you've ever uttered the words "My feet are killing me!" you need this book. This fun, concise guide will teach you how to pamper your feet and enjoy the total body benefits of good foot health—even when you're always on the go. With its easy-to-follow advice, it shows you how to soothe your aching feet to reduce stress, promote relaxation, and restore energy. So take the right step with *The Little Foot Care Book*.